Baking for the
Specific Carbohydrate Diet™

100 Grain-Free, Sugar-Free, Gluten-Free Recipes

Kathryn Anible

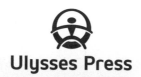

Ulysses Press

Published in the U.S. by
ULYSSES PRESS
P.O. Box 3440
Berkeley, CA 94703
www.ulyssespress.com

ISBN: 978-1-61243-489-6
Library of Congress Control Number: 2015937155

Printed in the United States by United Graphics Inc.
10 9 8 7 6 5 4 3 2 1

Acquisitions Editor: Casie Vogel
Managing Editor: Claire Chun
Project Editor: Alice Riegert
Editor: Susan Lang
Proofreader: Nancy Bell
Front cover and interior design/layout: what!design @ whatweb.com
Cover photos: plum and almond tart © Elena Shashkina/shutterstock.com; rye bread © AnjelikaGr/shutterstock.com; baking ingredients © Stock Rocket/shutterstock.com

Distributed by Publishers Group West

NOTE TO READERS: This book has been written and published strictly for informational and educational purposes only. It is not intended to serve as medical advice or to be any form of medical treatment. You should always consult your physician before altering or changing any aspect of your medical treatment and/or undertaking a diet regimen, including the guidelines as described in this book. Do not stop or change any prescription medications without the guidance and advice of your physician. Any use of the information in this book is made on the reader's good judgment after consulting with his or her physician and is the reader's sole responsibility. This book is not intended to diagnose or treat any medical condition and is not a substitute for a physician.

This book is independently authored and published and no sponsorship or endorsement of this book by, and no affiliation with, any trademarked brands or other products mentioned within is claimed or suggested. All trademarks that appear in ingredient lists and elsewhere in this book belong to their respective owners and are used here for informational purposes only. The authors and publishers encourage readers to patronize the quality brands mentioned and pictured in this book.

To my mom, Dennis, and friends for being my cheerleaders, supporters, and taste testers.

Contents

Chapter 6
Frostings and Sauces 123

Appendix: Essential SCD Recipes................................... 128

Conversions... 134

About the Author 137

Foreword

Dear SCD Bakers,

Thank you for joining me on this grand journey to better health. At times, it seems like an uphill trek with many obstacles, but it is worthwhile. I strongly believe that our health and happiness is directly linked to our choices about what we put into our bodies every day.

My goal with this book is to give you recipes to enjoy on every occasion—birthdays, holidays, or just brunch with friends—the same way that everybody else does. I want to change the implication that a diet is negatively restrictive. Guess what? You can be healthy and still eat cake, although I do recommend moderation.

As a private chef, I have spent years working with clients on their special diets, cooking meals (and occasionally desserts) that fit their specific needs. I have worked with many different types of diets, including gluten-free, vegan, soy-free, and even weight-gain diets. It gives me great pleasure to help relieve some of the pressure and struggle that can come with meal planning when you are on a diet.

My own family and several friends work at being gluten-free for various health reasons. Even while developing this book, I was able to help my mother, who had developed inflammation in her digestive tract, with her diet and in healing her gut.

Creating the recipes for this book was a challenge that I was happy to accept. At times, it seemed overwhelming, but I'm sure we have all felt stressed at some point when preparing food on SCD. Some recipes just didn't work and others had to be tested several times to make sure they were just right. I had baked goods everywhere in my house. I know, sounds tough, right? After months of baking, and giving my oven and mixer a good workout, I present these recipes to you. I'll admit, I have my favorites, such as Pineapple Upside-Down Cake (page 61) and Bacon Cheddar Bread (page 16). As you flip through the book and try some of the recipes, I hope that you find your own favorites that you can indulge in and that they help you heal.

I wish for you good food, good health, and much happiness!

Kathryn Anible

About SCD Baking

About the Specific Carbohydrate Diet

The Specific Carbohydrate Diet, or SCD, is a precise diet designed to help heal the digestive system. It is essential for those suffering from what can be debilitating disorders such as Crohn's disease, ulcerative colitis, irritable bowel syndrome, celiac disease, and other gastrointestinal ailments.

While this diet has helped many suffering from digestive disorders and other ailments, each individual is different and this diet might not be as effective for you as it is for some others. I recommend that you read *Breaking the Vicious Cycle* to get all of the information about SCD in your journey to better health and happiness and to consult with your doctor before beginning this diet.

The Specific Carbohydrate Diet was created by Drs. Sidney V. and Merrill P. Haas in 1951. It was designed to be a normal and nutritious diet, with a limit to the types of sugars and starches allowed. On the diet, only monosaccharides, the simplest form of carbohydrate, are allowed. If followed for a minimum of 1 year, the diet would allow some people to heal and then return to a normal way of eating without any digestive distress.

The SCD that is used today follows the writing of Elaine Gottschall in her book *Breaking the Vicious Cycle.* Her own daughter was diagnosed with ulcerative colitis at a young age and although they had tried many different medications and various treatments, nothing helped. In 1958, Dr. Sidney Haas prescribed this specific diet and within a short period Gottschall's daughter was able to stop taking medication and, remarkably, became free of all symptoms within 2 years. Elaine Gottschall wanted to learn more about the diet that cured her daughter and to share it with anyone whom it might help. She went on to study biology, cellular biology, and nutritional biochemistry, focusing her studies on the effects of sugar on the digestive system and the effects of inflammatory bowel disease on the intestinal walls.

Foods Allowed on the SCD

	Allowed	Not Allowed
Beans and Legumes	Black beans, kidney beans, lentils, lima beans, split peas, navy beans, peanuts	Any other bean, including chickpeas or garbanzo beans, fava beans, soy, and cannellini beans
Nuts and Seeds	All nuts, sesame seeds, sunflower seeds	Chia seeds, flax seeds, hemp seeds
Fats and Oils	All naturally occurring fats and oils	
Herbs and Spices	All are allowed	Anything that might have anti-caking agents in it; anything with the listing of "other spices" Avoid premade spice mixtures
Sweeteners	Honey, fruits, fruit juices, and saccharin	Table sugar, brown sugar, molasses, agave, stevia, or any other sweetener
Dairy and Eggs	Eggs, butter, SCD Yogurt, dry curd cottage cheese (DCCC), aged cheeses	Soft cheeses, milk, cream, half and half, cream cheese, cottage cheese (that is not dry curd)

Fruit	All fresh fruits, unsweetened frozen fruit, unsweetened dried fruit	No fruits that are canned, stored in syrup, or processed with sugar
Vegetables	Non-starchy vegetables, such as green beans, squash, carrots, peas, and spinach	Any starchy vegetables, such as potatoes, corn, , yams, sweet potatoes, and any mucilaginous vegetables, such as okra
Meats, Fish, and Poultry	All fresh meats, fish, and poultry; fish canned in oil or water	No processed or smoked meats, fish, or poultry; no additives, no added sugar

Baking on the SCD

While the Specific Carbohydrate Diet is strict, it is also very nutritious and balanced—yet can still be fun and full of sweet treats just like the goodies you already know and love. Baking seems like a challenge at first, as all-purpose flour, baking powder (as it has anti-caking agents), sugar, and yeast (because it promotes bacterial growth in the gut) are not allowed. But don't be discouraged. Instead, you can use nut and coconut flours, with eggs and baking soda as leaveners, and honey and dates as sweeteners.

A note about baking with SCD ingredients: Many of the ingredients are considered very advanced. Try each new ingredient slowly and see how you react. If you are baking for someone following SCD, make sure that person is able to tolerate each of the ingredients listed in the recipe, namely honey, nuts, eggs, and dates.

Pantry and Refrigerator Recommendations

Here are some of the foods I recommend keeping on hand for SCD baking. Some are specialty items that you will need to purchase online or at health food stores, and others you will come across easily.

Blanched Almond Flour

Blanched almond flour is the most popular nut flour in SCD baking, as it is the most widely available, is the most affordable and creates the best texture. Almonds are more easily digested when they are blanched and the fibrous skin is removed. You can substitute other nut flours for almond flour if you find that you cannot tolerate almonds, but keep in mind that a different nut flour will change the color and texture of a baked good.

Many brands of almond flour are available, with Bob's Red Mill being the most popular. If you plan on doing a lot of baking, check out Wellbee's (www.wellbees.com) or Tropical Traditions (www.tropicaltraditions.com), where you can buy almond flour in bulk. Both of these brands make their own blanched almond flour that is finely ground and creates a very nice texture, similar to all-purpose flour, in baked goods.

Coconut Flour

Coconut flour is used in combination with nut flour in many recipes throughout this book. It helps to reduce the denseness of some baked goods and creates a texture that more closely resembles baked goods made with all-purpose flour.

Again, many brands are available, but Tropical Traditions coconut flour seems to have the finest grind, which makes for a smoother, finer crumb in baked goods.

Honey

Honey is the main sweetener used in the recipes in this book. The color of the honey affects the color of the baked good. If you use a lighter colored honey, your baked good will be lighter in color, and a darker honey will produce a darker baked good. Keep in mind that some honeys are much sweeter than others, and you can only know by tasting them. Good sources of honey that you can taste test are farmer's markets. Be aware that honey caramelizes more quickly than sugar, so keep an eye on your baked goods and sauces when baking or cooking them.

Dates

With so many varieties and such a wide range of sweetness, dates make a very good addition to many baked goods. They add flavor, color, and, in some cases, texture. Whole California dates are allowed on SCD. You can find them in grocery stores and in big box retail stores, such as Costco. If you live in a warm climate, you may also find them at farmer's markets.

Pure Vanilla Extract

Some extracts contain fructose and other additives. SCD allows only for pure extracts with no additives. Penzy's Spices (www.penzys.com) is one brand that has been confirmed as SCD compliant. You can also make your own vanilla extract (as well as other kinds of extracts); see page 132.

SCD Yogurt

This is an ingredient that you must make yourself. It is mostly hands-off and requires little more than 24 hours before it is ready. You can find directions on page 129. SCD Yogurt is unique in that it ferments at 110°F for 24 hours, which allows the yogurt cultures to consume all of the lactose sugar. The yogurt can be stored in your refrigerator for up to one week.

Nut Milk

This is another ingredient that is best if you make it yourself. Commercially produced nut milks, like almond milk, usually have gums and thickeners added for a creamier texture and to prevent separation. Nut milk is very easy to make and requires only a few minutes of work. You can find a detailed recipe on page 128. The milk will store in the refrigerator for up to one week.

Coconut Milk

Coconut milk can be made at home if you have access to fresh coconut or unsweetened dried coconut flakes. You can find a recipe on page 130. If you don't have access to either of those ingredients, you may have to purchase coconut milk at the grocery store or online. A coconut milk that doesn't have any added gums or thickeners can be tricky to find, but there are some trusted brands available. Arroy-D carries both coconut milk and coconut cream without any added ingredients. It is available in some Asian markets and on Amazon.com.

Eggs

Eggs play a very big role in SCD baking. They act as a binder and leavening agent while also adding flavor and color to baked goods. For the best results, be sure to use the freshest eggs available to you.

Baking Soda

Baking soda is the leavening agent of choice when it comes to baking on SCD. Use the freshest baking soda that you can find, as time degrades this ingredient's effectiveness. Once the baking soda is open, be sure to store it in an airtight container to avoid it absorbing other flavors. Check the expiration label on your baking soda before using it in any recipe.

Other Essential Pantry and Refrigerated Items

- Cocoa butter (available online and in some specialty food stores)

- Coconut oil

- Olive oil

- Nuts and legal seeds

- Gelatin (unflavored)

- Unsalted butter

- Cheeses (SCD-allowed cheeses only)

- Fresh or frozen fruit (no sugar added)

Suggested Equipment

Some appliances make baking a little easier and quicker, but it's okay if you don't have all of the equipment on this list. A hand mixer or a large spoon or whisk and some elbow grease can definitely do the job of a stand mixer—and the same implements can stand in for a food processor.

- Stand mixer
- Food processor with shredder attachment or a box grater
- Blender
- 9-inch pie plate
- Two 9-inch cake pans
- Muffin tin
- Two 4 × 8-inch loaf pans
- Two baking sheets
- One 12 × 16-inch sheet pan
- One 7 × 11-inch baking dish
- 9 × 9-inch baking dish
- 9 × 13-inch baking dish
- Six 4-ounce ramekins
- Four 6-ounce ramekins
- Cake tester or toothpicks
- Parchment paper
- Plastic wrap
- Cutting board
- Paring knife
- Whisk
- Rubber spatula
- Microplane or zester
- Measuring cups
- Measuring spoons
- Rolling pin

Tips for Modifying Other Baking Recipes

Having a baking book filled with recipes that are designed specifically for your diet makes life so much easier, but sometimes there is a recipe from your pre-diet days that you just can't forget and would like to modify to fit your diet. At first, modifying recipes can seem daunting, but with a little practice, it gets easier. The only real way to know if something will work is to try it. These tips will put you on the right track.

Honey

Much sweeter than sugar, honey is the primary sweetener used in SCD baked goods. When using honey in place of sugar, reduce the amount to a quarter or a third of the amount of sugar called for in the original recipe. For instance, if a recipe calls for 1 cup of sugar, use ¼ or ⅓ cup of honey. Because honey adds a great deal of moisture, also reduce the amount of wet ingredients or add a little coconut flour to achieve the desired texture.

Date Paste

Different varieties of dates have different sweetness levels, so make sure to taste your dates before using them. Most dates will make a paste that is very near the sweetness of sugar, and using a 1 to 1 substitution of date paste for sugar should work. Since date paste adds more moisture to your baked goods, reduce the amount of other liquids like oil or milk, or add a little coconut flour, 1 teaspoon at a time, to the recipe to compensate. Date paste can sometimes be used as an egg substitute in baked goods, like in cookies. You can find a recipe for homemade date paste on page 131.

Blanched Almond Flour

Almond flour can be used in a 1 to 1 substitution for all-purpose flour in almost all recipes. It does tend to be a bit denser, so use a combination of almond flour and coconut flour in recipes when you want a finer crumb and a lighter product. For 1 cup of all-purpose flour, try ½ cup almond flour mixed with 2 tablespoons coconut flour. You may add more almond or coconut flour to the batter while mixing, if you find that the batter is much looser than the original recipe.

Coconut Flour

Coconut flour is very absorbent, so you can use much less of it: about ¼ cup per 1 cup of all-purpose flour. Using coconut flour exclusively, instead of almond flour, is possible, but the volume of the batter and baked goods will be much less than in the original recipe. Coconut flour creates a finer, looser crumb, which can sometimes result in a baked good that falls apart easily.

Baking Soda

Baking soda is a quick-rising leavener that also adds tenderness. It is about four times more potent than baking powder. Using too much of it can result in a baked good that rises very high and then falls flat as it continues to bake. Using ½ to 1 teaspoon will usually be enough to help a batter rise. To react, baking soda needs an acid, such as dry curd cottage cheese, yogurt, or honey. Because the reaction is immediate, the batter should be placed into the oven very soon after mixing together the acid ingredient with the baking soda.

Chapter 1
Breads and Crackers

Sandwich Bread

Bread is one of the household staples that make a busy life easier. You can pop a couple of slices into the toaster for a quick breakfast or throw together a sandwich for a fast and healthy lunch. This bread rises much like traditional breads and the crust is firm. It holds together when sliced and has a nice neutral flavor. Any leftovers can be made into croutons or bread pudding.

Makes: 1 loaf

1 cup almond or cashew butter

1 tablespoon coconut flour

5 large eggs, room temperature

1 teaspoon honey

1 teaspoon baking soda

¼ teaspoon salt

1 teaspoon apple cider vinegar

Preheat the oven to 350°F. Line a 4 × 8-inch loaf pan with parchment paper, and spray with vegetable oil.

Mix together all of the ingredients, except the vinegar. Once all of the ingredients are thoroughly combined, add the vinegar, mix quickly, and pour the batter into the prepared loaf pan.

Place the pan on the middle rack in the oven. Bake for 30 to 35 minutes, or until a cake tester inserted into the center comes out clean.

Sandwich Flatbread

This is a basic sandwich flatbread, similar to a tortilla but thicker. I love to toast two of these flatbreads and put a scrambled egg and avocado in between them for a breakfast sandwich. They also can be used like thinner versions of hamburger buns.

Makes: 4 flatbreads

1¼ cups blanched almond flour

¼ cup olive oil or coconut oil

1 large egg, room temperature

½ teaspoon salt

Preheat the oven to 350°F. Line two baking sheets with parchment paper.

Mix together all of the ingredients. Divide the dough into four equal portions. Form one portion into a ball, place on the baking sheet, and cover loosely with plastic wrap. Gently flatten the dough with your hands or a rolling pin until about ½ inch thick and 6 inches in diameter. Continue with the remaining dough. Place two flatbreads on each baking sheet.

Bake for 8 to 10 minutes or until the edges begin to brown.

Bacon Cheddar Bread

Bacon and cheese! What could be better? For breakfast, toast a slice of this bread and serve with eggs on top. Slather on mayonnaise, and pile on tomatoes and lettuce for a BLT lunch. The bread has little flecks of bacon and cheese throughout, giving every bite a delicious burst of flavor.

Makes: 1 loaf

1 cup nut butter, such as almond or cashew

1 tablespoon coconut flour

½ teaspoon baking soda

¼ teaspoon salt

5 large eggs, room temperature

1 cup shredded cheddar plus 2 tablespoons, divided

¾ cup chopped bacon (about 10 slices), divided

Preheat the oven to 350°F. Line a 4 × 8-inch loaf pan with parchment paper, and spray with vegetable oil.

Mix together the nut butter, flour, baking soda, salt, and eggs. Add 1 cup of the cheese and ½ cup of the bacon, stirring to combine. Pour the batter into the prepared pan. Sprinkle the top with the remaining cheese and bacon.

Bake for 30 to 35 minutes, or until a cake tester inserted in the center comes out clean.

Calzone

Mmm, pizza pockets! This is a healthy way to satisfy your junk food cravings. My favorites are the classic tomato, basil, and cheese combo or sautéed mushrooms and spinach with cheese. For a Southwestern flavor, fill the pockets with cooked and seasoned ground beef, sautéed peppers and onions, and some cumin.

Makes: 2 large calzones

2 cups blanched almond flour

3 large eggs, room temperature, divided

¼ cup (½ stick) unsalted butter, chilled and cut into cubes

1 teaspoon baking soda

½ teaspoon garlic powder (optional)

½ teaspoon dried oregano or 1 teaspoon fresh (optional)

1 cup shredded cheese, such as Parmesan, provolone, or dry curd cottage cheese (DCCC)

1 cup cooked filling, such as ground meats or vegetables

½ to 1 teaspoon seasoning of choice, such as garlic, basil, or onion

2 tablespoons grated Parmesan (optional)

1 cup tomato sauce, warmed (optional)

Preheat the oven to 350°F. Combine the flour, two of the eggs, and the butter, baking soda, and garlic powder and oregano, if using. Mix until the dough comes together, then divide it in half.

Roll out each half between sheets of parchment paper until about ¼ to ½ inch thick and in the shape of a circle, about 12 to 14 inches in diameter. Place the parchment with the rolled out dough onto a baking sheet. Remove the top layer of parchment and divide the filling between the dough circles, placing it just off-center. Grab the two corners of the parchment paper on the side that does not have filling on it, and fold the dough over the filling. Crimp the edges of the dough to seal it. Beat the remaining egg, and brush the egg wash over the top of the calzones. Sprinkle with Parmesan, if using.

Bake for 10 to 15 minutes, or until the top and edges begin to brown. If using tomato sauce for dipping, serve it on the side.

Flatbread or Pizza Crust

This is an incredibly versatile and delicious recipe. Season this with your favorite herbs and bake it for a yummy flatbread. If you roll it out a little thinner, you can top it with your favorite sauce and pizza toppings for a scrumptious dinner or snack. Kids love it, and it's easy to make. There's no need to wait for yeast to rise, because in this recipe the eggs do all the work.

Flatbread is delicious with your favorite salad served on top, or with some pesto and fresh tomatoes.

Makes: One 12-inch flatbread or pizza

1 cup blanched almond flour

¼ cup coconut flour

½ teaspoon salt

¼ teaspoon baking soda

1 teaspoon herbs and spices, such as basil, oregano, thyme, parsley, and garlic

½ cup (1 stick) unsalted butter, softened

2 large eggs, room temperature

Preheat the oven to 350°F. Line a baking sheet with parchment paper.

Mix together all of the ingredients, until well combined. Using your hands or a rolling pin, flatten the dough on the baking sheet, until about ½ inch thick and circular or square shaped.

IF MAKING FLATBREAD: Bake for 10 to 15 minutes, or until the edges have browned slightly.

IF MAKING PIZZA: Bake the crust for 5 minutes, add the sauce and toppings, and bake for an additional 10 to 12 minutes, or until the edges are browned.

Turn It into Breadsticks

Alternatively, this can be made into breadsticks, if you roll the dough out to ¾ inch thick. Back for 10 to 15 minutes and then slice into breadsticks.

Garlic Parmesan Bread

I love cheesy garlic bread, and this one hits the spot. You can add more or less garlic, depending on how much you like it. Use garlic powder for a more powerful garlic flavor or fresh garlic for a milder flavor. Serve this bread with an Italian meal with lots of tomato sauce.

Makes: 1 loaf

1 cup nut butter

1 tablespoon coconut flour

5 large eggs

½ teaspoon baking soda

¼ teaspoon salt

6 cloves garlic, minced, or 1½ teaspoons garlic powder

½ cup shredded Parmesan plus more for sprinkling on top

Preheat the oven to 350°F. Line a 4 × 8-inch loaf pan with parchment paper and spray with vegetable oil.

Mix together the nut butter, flour, eggs, baking soda, salt, garlic, and ½ cup of the Parmesan. Pour the batter into the loaf pan, and sprinkle some Parmesan on top. Bake for 30 to 35 minutes, or until a cake tester inserted in the center comes out clean.

Cheese Dinner Rolls

This dinner roll is so delicious and addictive! It makes an excellent breakfast sandwich and is great for dipping into a little tomato sauce.

Makes: 12 large rolls or 16 small rolls

1½ cups blanched almond flour

1 teaspoon baking soda

½ teaspoon salt

½ cup (1 stick) unsalted butter, room temperature

1 large egg, room temperature

1 cup shredded cheese, such as cheddar or Parmesan

Preheat the oven to 350°F. Prepare a baking sheet by lining it with parchment paper or spraying the surface with vegetable oil.

In a bowl, mix together the flour, baking soda, and salt. Add the butter and the egg, mixing until completely combined. Stir in the cheese, then refrigerate the dough for 10 minutes. After 10 minutes, remove the dough and divide it into equal portions, rolling them into balls about 1 to 2 inches in diameter.

Bake for 15 to 20 minutes, or until the edges begin to turn light brown.

Turn It into Breadsticks

If you form the dough into a log shape instead of balls, you can get breadsticks instead of rolls.

Banana Bread

Here's a tasty way to use up overripe bananas and get your dose of potassium. This bread is also a delicious way to start the morning. Share a loaf with a friend or turn the leftovers into bread pudding.

Makes: 2 loaves, or 16 to 20 servings

¾ cup coconut flour

2 teaspoons baking soda

½ teaspoon salt

3 medium ripe bananas

6 tablespoons unsalted butter, softened

5 large eggs, room temperature

1 teaspoon pure vanilla extract

2 teaspoons apple cider vinegar

¼ cup chopped nuts (optional)

Preheat the oven to 325°F. Prepare two 4 inch by 8 inch loaf pans by lining them with parchment paper and spraying with vegetable oil.

In a bowl, whisk together the flour, baking soda, and salt. In a separate bowl, beat the bananas, butter, and honey. To the banana mixture, add the eggs one at a time, mixing between additions, then add the vanilla, vinegar, and nuts, if using. Mix everything together until it is well combined. Add the flour mixture to the banana mixture, and mix until just combined.

Divide the batter evenly between the prepared loaf pans. Bake for 50 to 60 minutes, or until a cake tester inserted in the center comes out clean.

Irish Soda Bread

There are many variations of soda bread. This version is slightly sweet and contains dried fruit, making it equally good for breakfast or a sweet snack. It is delicious toasted and slathered with butter.

Makes: 1 loaf, 8 to 10 servings

2 cups blanched almond flour

¼ cup coconut flour

1 teaspoon baking soda

½ teaspoon salt

¼ cup Date Paste (page 131)

1 large egg

½ cup SCD Yogurt (page 129)

2 tablespoons unsalted butter, room temperature

1 teaspoon orange zest

¼ cup dried, unsulfured, unsweetened currants or raisins

Preheat the oven to 350°F. Line a baking sheet with parchment paper.

In a bowl, whisk together the flours, baking soda, and salt, making sure there are no clumps. In a separate bowl, combine the date paste, egg, yogurt, butter, and orange zest. Add the date mixture to the flour mixture, and stir together. Fold in the currants or raisins. Form the dough into a ball, and place it on the prepared baking sheet.

Bake for 40 to 45 minutes, or until the crust is golden and a tester inserted in the center comes out clean. Allow to cool before slicing.

Cinnamon Raisin Bread

Baking this bread will make your whole house smell of cinnamon. This is a kid and adult favorite, so good luck trying to keep any of this loaf in your home for long!

Makes: 1 loaf, 8 to 10 servings

FOR THE FILLING

⅓ cup honey

1 tablespoon ground cinnamon

¼ cup raisins

FOR THE BREAD

1 cup nut butter

4 large eggs

2 tablespoons honey

1 tablespoon coconut flour

1 teaspoon baking soda

¼ teaspoon ground cinnamon

Preheat the oven to 350°F. Line a 4 × 8-inch loaf pan with parchment paper and spray with vegetable oil.

In a small bowl, mix together the ingredients for the filling, and set aside. In a separate bowl, food processor, or stand mixer, mix together all of the ingredients for the bread. Pour a third of the bread mixture into the loaf pan, then drizzle in a third of the filling. Continue adding the bread mixture and the filling in thirds, finishing with the filling on top. The filling will sink during baking.

Bake for 30 to 35 minutes, or until the edges are browned and a tester inserted in the center comes out clean. Allow to cool slightly before serving. This bread can remain at room temperature for three days or in the refrigerator for up to a week.

Pumpkin Bread

When autumn rolls around, I like to bake with pumpkin—and that includes making this flavorful bread. Moist and delicious, it smells like cinnamon and nutmeg while it bakes. If you have trouble finding pure pumpkin, you can use a fresh sugar pumpkin or butternut squash. Enjoy this bread on its own or top it with the Basic Buttercream Frosting, page 124, to make it a treat.

Makes: 2 loaves, or 16 to 20 servings

1 cup coconut flour

1½ cups almond flour

1 tablespoon baking soda

½ teaspoon salt

1 teaspoon ground cinnamon

1 teaspoon ground nutmeg

½ teaspoon ground cloves

½ teaspoon ground allspice

½ cup (1 stick) butter, room temperature

1 cup honey

5 large eggs, room temperature

1 cup pure pumpkin puree

1 teaspoon pure vanilla extract

½ cup dry curd cottage cheese (DCCC) or SCD Yogurt (page 129)

½ cup raisins (optional)

½ cup nuts (optional)

Preheat the oven to 350°F. Line two 4 inch by 8 inch loaf pans with parchment paper and spray with vegetable oil.

In a medium bowl, whisk together the flours, baking soda, salt, and spices, making sure there are no clumps. In a separate bowl, whip the butter until very light in color. Add the honey, and continue mixing. Add the eggs one at a time, incorporating each before adding the next egg. Mix in the pumpkin, vanilla, and cottage cheese or yogurt.

Add half of the flour mixture to the pumpkin mixture, and combine until incorporated. Then add the other half of the mixture, and stir in the raisins and nuts, if using. Continue mixing until fully incorporated. Divide the batter between the loaf pans.

Bake for 1 hour, or until the bread is browned on the edges and the center is set, or when a tester inserted in the center comes out clean.

Make It Into Muffins

This can easily be made into muffins. Simply divide the batter into 24 muffin cups and bake for 30 to 40 minutes

Gingerbread

During the fall and winter months, when the air gets cooler and cold and flu season is upon us, this bread is wonderful to have around. Ginger has been known to help with nausea and indigestion, while cinnamon is an antimicrobial. This could be the key to keeping you healthy during the winter. Okay, maybe it doesn't have those superpowers, but it will make your mouth happy and it makes a great gift during the holidays. Serve this gingerbread with a little butter, Basic Buttercream Frosting (page 124).

Makes: 1 loaf or 8 to 10 servings

1 cup nut butter

4 large eggs

¼ cup honey

¼ cup Date Paste (page 131)

1 teaspoon baking soda

½ teaspoon salt

1 tablespoon ground ginger

1 teaspoon ground cinnamon

¼ teaspoon ground nutmeg

⅛ teaspoon ground cloves

Preheat the oven to 350°F. Line a 4 × 8-inch loaf pan with parchment paper or oil the insides.

In a bowl, mix together all of the ingredients until well combined. Pour the batter into the loaf pan.

Bake for 30 to 40 minutes, or until a tester inserted in the center of the loaf comes out clean. Allow to cool slightly before serving.

Coconut Cream Biscuits

These amazing biscuits are so good with saucy dinners, like chicken with gravy or zoodles with tomato sauce. They are also delicious with butter or jam and great for breakfast. The coconut cream gives them a rich flavor.

Makes: 8 to 10 biscuits

1 cup blanched almond flour

¼ cup coconut flour

1 teaspoon baking soda

½ teaspoon salt

¾ cup Coconut Cream (page 130)

2 teaspoons honey

Preheat the oven to 400°F. Line a baking sheet with parchment paper or spray with oil.

Whisk together the flours, baking soda, and salt. Add the coconut cream and honey, mixing until just combined. For each biscuit, drop ¼ cup of the batter onto the baking sheet, leaving 2 inches between biscuits.

Bake for 12 to 15 minutes, until the edges of the biscuits are browned and a tester inserted in the center of a biscuit comes out clean. Serve warm or at room temperature.

 EGG-FREE

Peach Bread

Peach season lasts only a few short weeks. Why not try to get as much of the sweet, juicy fruit as you can? This bread has just a hint of sweetness, most it from the peaches. It is moist and makes as good a breakfast as it does a light dessert. You can use nectarines in place of peaches. White peaches and white nectarines are lower in acidity and easier for some people to digest.

Makes: 1 loaf or 8 to 10 servings

¾ cup nut butter, such as almond or cashew

4 large eggs

¼ cup honey

1½ cups sliced peaches (about 3 small or 1½ large), divided

½ teaspoon ground cinnamon

½ teaspoon baking soda

Preheat the oven to 350°F. Line a 4 × 8-inch loaf pan with parchment paper and spray with vegetable oil.

In a food processor, add the nut butter, the eggs, honey, 1 cup of the peaches, the cinnamon, and the baking soda. Mix on low for about 1 minute, until all of the ingredients come together and are well blended. Pour the batter into the prepared loaf pan. Layer the remaining peach slices on top of the batter. They will sink into the bread as it bakes.

Bake for 20 to 25 minutes, or until a cake tester inserted in the center comes out clean. Allow to cool before slicing.

Almond Crackers

Crunchy and a little salty, these crackers are great on their own or for scooping up dips. You can make these crackers as big or as small as desired.

Makes: About 45 crackers

2 cups blanched almond flour

2 tablespoons ice water

1 tablespoon coconut oil or olive oil

½ teaspoon salt

Preheat the oven to 350°F.

In a bowl, mix together all of the ingredients until combined. Roll out the dough between two sheets of parchment paper, until rectangular and about ¼ inch thick. Remove the top sheet of parchment paper and place the bottom sheet, with the dough, on a baking sheet.

Bake for 5 minutes, then take out the cookie sheet and slice the dough into 1" by 2" rectangles. Return to the oven and continue baking for an additional 10 to 15 minutes, or until the edges start to brown. Allow the crackers to cool completely on the baking sheet. Once cooled, store in an airtight container.

 EGG-FREE

Cheese Crackers

A salty, crunchy, and kid-friendly snack, these cheese crackers are simple to make. You can easily double the recipe so you're sure to have plenty of snacks on hand.

Makes: About 45 crackers

1 cup freshly shredded cheese, such as cheddar or Parmesan

¼ cup (½ stick) unsalted butter, chilled

¾ teaspoon salt

1 cup blanched almond flour

2 tablespoons ice water

Preheat the oven to 350°F.

In a food processor combine the cheese, butter, salt, and flour. Add the ice water 1 tablespoon at a time, and process until the dough comes together, about 5 to 10 seconds.

Between two sheets of parchment paper, roll the dough into a rectangle until even and about ¼ inch thick. Remove the top sheet of parchment and place the bottom sheet, with the dough, on a cookie sheet.

Bake in the oven for 7 minutes, then take out the baking sheet and slice the dough into 1" by 2" rectangles. Return to the oven, and continue baking for an additional 10 to 15 minutes, or until the edges start to brown. Allow the crackers to cool completely on the baking sheet. Store in an airtight container.

 EGG-FREE

Cheese Crisps

These cheese crackers couldn't be easier to make or more delicious. They are also incredibly addictive. They'll satisfy your craving for salty snacks.

Makes: 12 crackers

1 cup shredded cheese, such as Parmesan or cheddar

½ teaspoon herbs and spices of choice (optional)

Preheat the oven to 350°F. Line a baking sheet with parchment paper.

Toss the cheese with herbs and spices, if using. Using a tablespoon, portion the cheese onto the parchment-lined baking sheet, leaving 2 to 3 inches between portions. Bake for 5 to 8 minutes, or until the cheese has bubbled for a couple of minutes. Take the pan out of the oven, and allow the crisps to cool completely before removing them from the pan.

Flavor Suggestions

Rosemary Parmesan

Cayenne cheddar

Dill Havarti

Basil, oregano, and rosemary provolone

 EGG-FREE

Veggie Chips

Craving a salty, crunchy snack? These chips will hit the spot, and they are a quick, delicious way to get veggie servings and fiber. The best results come from using a mandoline to slice the vegetables, so they bake evenly and you don't end up with any overcooked chips, but a good sharp knife can do the trick as well. The best SCD-friendly veggies to use for this recipe are zucchini, summer squash, carrots, beets, and turnips.

Makes: About ¾ cup chips

1½ cups thinly sliced vegetables	2 teaspoons olive oil
¼ teaspoon salt	1 teaspoon herbs and spices of choice

Preheat the oven to 375°F. Prepare a baking sheet by lining it with parchment paper.

Lay the vegetable slices in a single layer on a towel or paper towel. Sprinkle with the salt, and let sit for about 5 minutes. Then gently toss with the oil and the herbs and spices. Place in a single layer on the parchment paper. Bake for 15 to 20 minutes, rotating after 10 minutes. After 15 minutes, start checking the chips every 2 to 3 minutes and remove any that have begun to brown. They may still be soft, but should crisp up as they cool. Once cooled completely, store in an airtight container.

Flavor Suggestions

ITALIAN: Garlic powder, oregano, basil

CREOLE: Paprika, thyme, chili powder, cayenne

MEXICAN: Cumin, garlic, oregano, chili powder, paprika

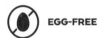 **EGG-FREE**

Graham Crackers

These are mildly sweet and crunchy crackers that both children and adults will enjoy. Try them with a little nut butter spread and sliced bananas on top.

Makes: 12 large crackers

1 cup blanched almond flour

2 tablespoons honey

¼ cup Date Paste (page 131)

2 tablespoons unsalted butter, softened

½ teaspoon ground cinnamon

⅛ teaspoon salt

Preheat the oven to 350°F. Line a baking sheet with parchment paper.

Mix together all of the ingredients until well combined. Using a spatula, evenly spread the dough over the parchment paper until it is about ¼ inch thick and forms a rectangle about 10 inches by 14 inches. Cut the dough with a rolling pizza cutter.

Bake for 12 to 15 minutes, or until the edges begin to brown. Allow the crackers to cool completely before breaking them into individual pieces. Store in an airtight container.

Graham Cracker Crust

You can use these crackers to make a graham cracker crust. Break the crackers into crumbs, and combine them with 2 tablespoons of melted butter. Press the mixture into a pie dish, refrigerate for 30 minutes, and then pour your filling into the crust.

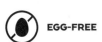 **EGG-FREE**

Chapter 2
Muffins and Cakes

Yellow Cake

Who doesn't love cake? This recipe can be made into a show-stopping layer cake for birthdays, following the directions in the sidebar on the following page. The key to a light cake is gently folding the whipped egg whites into the cake batter.

Makes: 16 to 20 servings

1 cup (2 sticks) unsalted butter, room temperature

1 cup honey

½ cup cashew butter

4 large eggs, separated, room temperature

½ cup SCD Yogurt (page 129)

1 tablespoon pure vanilla extract

2 cups blanched almond flour

1½ teaspoons baking soda

½ teaspoon salt

Preheat the oven to 350°F. Line a 9-inch cake pan with parchment paper and butter the sides.

Beat the butter until light and creamy. Mix in the honey and cashew butter. Add the egg yolks one at a time, mixing between additions. Next, incorporate the yogurt and the vanilla. In a separate bowl, whisk together the flour, baking soda, and salt. In a clean bowl, whip the egg whites until soft peaks form.

Pour the butter mixture into the flour mixture, and stir until combined. Fold the whipped whites into the batter, incorporating a third of the whites at a time, until there are no visible whites. Divide the batter evenly between the two cake pans.

Bake for 35 to 45 minutes, or until a tester inserted in the center comes out clean. Allow to cool completely before removing from the pans. Store unfrosted cakes covered in the refrigerator for up to two weeks, or frosted for up to one week.

TIP: To line the bottom of a cake pan, trace the bottom of the pan on parchment paper and cut out the circle with scissors.

Make a Layer Cake

To make a layered cake, slice the tops off of the baked cakes to make them even. I like to use a combination of Fruit Sauce (page 127) and Basic Buttercream Frosting (page 124). Spread a little fruit sauce and buttercream over the bottom layer, then put on the top layer and cover with frosting. I love to add flowers for decoration.

Lemon Poppy Seed Muffins

Make these muffins for breakfast or brunch. They have such a bright flavor, they're like bites of sunshine. I like to feature them in an Easter or Mother's Day brunch buffet.

Makes: 12 servings

1 cup nut butter

⅓ cup honey

4 large eggs, room temperature

½ teaspoon baking soda

½ teaspoon pure vanilla extract

2 tablespoons lemon zest

2 tablespoons fresh lemon juice or ½ teaspoon lemon extract

2 teaspoons poppy seeds

Preheat the oven to 350°F. Place paper liners in a muffin tin.

In a large bowl, mix together all of the ingredients. Pour about ¼ cup of batter into each muffin cup. Bake for 25 to 30 minutes, or until a cake tester inserted in the center of a muffin comes out clean. Carefully remove the muffins from the pan and allow them to cool. Once the muffins have cooled, store in airtight containers for up to one week at room temperature or two weeks refrigerated.

Orange Cake

Refreshing and delicious, this cake tastes a little like orange marmalade. Drizzle the cake with a little honey, and top it with some orange segments or raspberries for a showier dessert to share with guests.

Makes: 8 to 10 servings

1 cup blanched almond flour

¼ cup coconut flour

½ teaspoon baking soda

¼ teaspoon salt

4 large eggs, room temperature

⅓ cup honey

¼ cup (½ stick) unsalted butter, softened

¼ cup SCD Yogurt (page 129)

2 tablespoons fresh orange juice

zest of 1 orange

Preheat the oven to 350°F. Line a 9-inch cake pan with parchment paper and butter the sides.

In a bowl, whisk together the flours, baking soda, and salt, making sure there are no clumps. In a separate bowl, mix together the eggs, honey, butter, yogurt, orange juice, and orange zest. Add the egg mixture to the flour mixture, and stir to combine. Pour the batter into the prepared cake pan.

Bake for 20 to 25 minutes, or until a cake tester inserted in the center comes out clean. Allow the cake to cool completely before removing it from the pan. Store covered in the fridge for up to two weeks.

TIP: You can change the citrus in the recipe, if you prefer the flavor of lime, lemon, or grapefruit, but make sure to change both the juice and the zest.

Apple Cake

When I was growing up, autumn meant apples: everything from applesauce to stewed apples over pork roast. This cake is one more delectable way to enjoy apples. The spices in this cake smell marvelous and fill your home with the scent of cinnamon! Use your favorite apple variety or mix it up and use a pear instead!

Makes: 8 to 10 servings

1½ cups blanched almond flour

¼ cup coconut flour

1 teaspoon baking soda

¼ teaspoon salt

1 teaspoon ground cinnamon

⅛ teaspoon ground nutmeg

⅛ teaspoon ground cloves

¼ cup (½ stick) unsalted butter, softened

¼ cup applesauce

½ cup SCD Yogurt (page 129)

½ cup honey

2 large eggs, room temperature

1 teaspoon pure vanilla extract

1 large apple, peeled, cored, and cut into ¼-inch thick slices

Preheat the oven to 350°F. Line a 9-inch cake pan with parchment paper or butter the bottom and sides.

In a large bowl, whisk together the flours, baking soda, salt, and spices. In a food processor or stand mixer, combine the butter, applesauce, yogurt, honey, eggs, and vanilla. Pulse or mix until completely combined. Add the butter mixture to the flour mixture, and stir to combine. Pour the cake batter into the cake pan, and spread until even. Arrange the apple slices on top of the batter.

Bake for 30 to 35 minutes, or until a tester inserted in the center comes out clean. Allow to cool for at least 10 minutes before serving. Store covered in the fridge for up one week.

Lemon Pound Cake

Lemon pound cake is one of those delicious baked goods that makes a lovely afternoon snack, dessert, or gift. This cake is fragrant and citrusy, and, despite its name, light. The lightness comes from egg whites folded in at the end, and from allowing the cake to cool in the oven. Cooling in the oven prevents it from falling, which is a common occurrence with SCD baked goods. You can bake the cake in either a Bundt pan or two loaf pans. The oven temperature and baking time are the same.

Makes: 16 to 20 servings

1 cup (2 sticks) unsalted butter, softened

¾ cup honey

½ cup SCD Yogurt (page 129)

½ cup fresh lemon juice (about 3 large lemons)

2 tablespoons lemon zest

5 eggs, separated, room temperature

2 cups blanched almond flour

2 tablespoons coconut flour

1 teaspoon salt

1 teaspoon baking soda

Preheat the oven to 375°F. Prepare the Bundt pan by spraying it with oil or prepare the two 4 × 8-inch loaf pans by lining them with parchment paper and spraying them with oil.

In a bowl, mix together the butter and honey. Continue mixing while slowly adding the lemon juice, lemon zest, and the egg yolks, one yolk at a time. In another bowl, whisk together the flours, salt, and baking soda, making sure there are no clumps. In a separate bowl, whip the egg whites until soft peaks form. Add the flour mixture to the butter mixture, and stir to combine. Once the batter is well incorporated, fold the whipped whites into the batter, incorporating a third of the whites at a time, until there are no visible whites. Pour the batter into the prepared Bundt pan or loaf pans.

Bake for 10 minutes. Lower the oven temperature to 300°F, and continue to bake for 40 minutes. Turn the oven off, crack the oven door open, and leave the cake in the oven an additional 20 minutes. After 20 minutes, remove the cake and allow it to cool completely before slicing and serving. Store covered in the refrigerator for up to one week.

Sponge Cake

Light and fluffy, sponge cake can be turned into many other things. It can be a base for a trifle, or you can add jam and make a jelly roll. You can also cut this cake in half or quarters and make a very light, multilayer cake. Because it's baked in a sheet pan, the cake is very thin. For a thicker cake, you could use a smaller 12-inch or 9-inch cake pan, but remember to add 10 to 20 minutes to your baking time.

Makes: 1 thin sheet cake

1 cup blanched almond flour

½ teaspoon baking soda

¼ teaspoon salt

3 tablespoons SCD Yogurt (page 129) or dry curd cottage cheese (DCCC)

½ teaspoon pure vanilla extract

5 large eggs, room temperature

⅓ cup honey

Preheat the oven to 350°F. Line a 12 × 16-inch sheet pan with parchment paper and spray it with oil.

In a medium bowl, combine the flour, baking soda, and salt. In a separate bowl, whisk together the yogurt or DCCC, vanilla, eggs, and honey. Whisk until the eggs are completely combined. Add the egg mixture to the flour mixture, and mix until well combined. The batter will be very liquidy. Pour it into the prepared pan.

Bake for 20 to 25 minutes, or until the center is firm to the touch. Allow the cake to cool completely before removing it from the pan. Store the cake covered in the refrigerator for up to one week.

Microwave Mug Cake

A single-serving cake that is ready in less than 5 minutes and satisfies a sweet tooth? Yup! This cake is fluffy and warm right out of the microwave. It is delicious on its own, or add Fruit Sauce (page 127) and Coconut Cream (page 130) for extra decadence.

Makes: 1 serving

⅓ cup blanched almond flour

1 large egg

2 tablespoon honey

1 tablespoon dried fruit or nuts (optional)

¼ teaspoon pure vanilla extract or almond extract

⅛ teaspoon baking soda

⅛ teaspoon ground cinnamon (optional)

Mix all of the ingredients together in a coffee mug. Microwave on high for 90 seconds. The cake will rise above the edge of the cup but will not spill over. Serve immediately.

Black Bean "Chocolate" Cake

Not really chocolate, but cocoa butter is a good flavor substitute in this dark, fluffy cake that is airy and almost sponge-like, thanks to whipped egg whites and baking soda. Double the recipe to make a layer cake, and pair it with any frosting in this book for a decadent birthday cake.

Makes: 8 to 10 servings

½ cup cocoa butter, melted and cooled

1½ cups cooked black beans*

5 large eggs, separated, room temperature

⅓ cup honey

1½ teaspoons coffee extract

½ teaspoon baking soda

*To make beans SCD legal, soak in water overnight and then rinse before cooking them. Boil for about 15 minutes and then simmer for about 35 minutes, or until the beans are soft. Be sure to remove any scum that rises to the top.

Preheat the oven to 350°F. Line the bottom of a 9-inch square cake pan with parchment paper, and spray the sides with oil.

In a blender, combine the black beans, egg yolks, honey, coffee extract, and baking soda. Blend until the mixture is very smooth, 1 to 2 minutes. Pour the mixture into a bowl. Stir in the melted cocoa butter. In a separate bowl, beat the egg whites until soft peaks form. Fold the whipped whites into the batter, incorporating a third of the whites at a time, until there are no visible whites or lumps. Pour the batter into the prepared cake pan.

Bake for 35 to 45 minutes, or until a cake tester inserted in the center comes out clean. Allow the cake to cool before removing it from the pan and frosting it. Store covered in the refrigerator for up to one week.

Bacon, Egg, and Cheese Muffins

Want a super-simple breakfast that is fun to eat? This is the all-American breakfast in miniature. You can assemble these muffins the night before and bake them in the morning, or make them ahead of time and reheat them in the oven. Either way, they are a great grab-and-go breakfast option. You can use other hard cheeses besides cheddar, as long as they are SCD legal. This recipe calls for medium eggs, since large eggs overflow in standard muffin cups. If you have larger muffin cups, go ahead and use large eggs.

Makes: 6 servings

½ cup blanched almond flour

1 tablespoon plus ¼ cup shredded cheddar, divided

1 teaspoon unsalted butter

3 to 6 slices sugar-free bacon

6 medium eggs

Preheat the oven to 350°F. Prepare a muffin pan by spraying the cups with vegetable oil.

Mix together the flour, 1 tablespoon of the cheese, and the butter. Divide the mixture among six muffin cups, pressing about 1 heaping tablespoon into the bottom of each cup. Line the sides of the cups with a single layer of bacon, cutting the bacon if it is too long. Break 1 egg into each cup. If you prefer the eggs scrambled, beat them individually before adding them to the muffin cups. Sprinkle the remaining cheese on top.

Bake for 18 to 22 minutes, or just until the eggs are set. Serve hot. Store remaining muffins covered in the refrigerator for up to one week.

Apricot Cake

This looks a bit like an upside-down cake, but it doesn't require the effort of flipping the cake over. The fruit is placed on top, making the cake very easy to assemble. While there is a sweetness, the flavor is very mellow and the sweetness mostly comes from the apricots. The texture is light and spongy, making this cake just right for brunch or as a summer dessert with an apricot or blackberry Fruit Sauce, page 127. For a slightly sweeter cake, substitute peaches or nectarines for the apricots.

Makes: 8 to 10 servings

1 cup (2 sticks) unsalted butter, softened

¼ cup SCD Yogurt (page 129)

1 cup Date Paste (page 131)

3 large eggs, separated, room temperature

1 teaspoon pure vanilla extract

2 cups blanched almond flour

1 teaspoon baking soda

6 to 8 apricots, cut in half, pits removed

Preheat the oven to 350°F. Line the bottom of a 9-inch cake pan with parchment paper, and butter the sides.

Mix together the butter, yogurt, date paste, egg yolks, and vanilla. In a separate bowl, whisk together the flour and the baking soda. Whip the egg whites until soft peaks form. Stir the butter mixture into the flour mixture until well combined. Fold the whipped whites into the batter, incorporating a third of the whites at a time, until there are no visible whites. Pour the batter into the prepared cake pan. Arrange the apricot halves, cut side down, on top of the batter. They will sink slightly during baking.

Bake for 35 to 40 minutes, or until a cake tester inserted in the center comes out clean. Let cool completely before serving. The cake can be stored, covered, in the refrigerator for up to one week.

Carrot Cake

Moist and flavorful as carrot cake is, no wonder this dessert is a favorite for birthdays! Once the cake is topped with Basic Buttercream Frosting (page 124), no one will suspect that it is grain-free.

Makes: 8 to 10 servings

1 pound carrots, peeled and grated

1½ cups blanched almond flour

½ cup coconut flour

1¾ teaspoon baking soda

½ teaspoon salt

1¼ teaspoon ground cinnamon

½ teaspoon ground nutmeg

⅛ teaspoon ground cloves

1 cup honey

4 large eggs

1 cup vegetable oil or coconut oil

1 teaspoon apple cider vinegar or lemon juice

¼ cup raisins (optional)

¼ cup chopped nuts (optional)

Basic Buttercream Frosting (page 124)

Preheat the oven to 350°F. Oil one 9-inch square cake pan.

In a large bowl, stir together the carrots, flours, baking soda, salt, and spices. In a separate bowl, mix together the honey, eggs, oil, and vinegar. Add the egg mixture to the carrot mixture, and stir until just combined. Fold in the raisins and nuts, if using. Pour the batter into the prepared pan or pans.

Bake for 40 to 50 minutes, or until a cake tester inserted comes out clean. Allow to cool completely, at least 2 hours, before frosting the cake. To make it a layer cake, carefully slice through the center of the cake to make two 9-inch cakes. Store the cake covered in the refrigerator for up to one week.

Coconut Cake

A Southern favorite, coconut cake is an elegant addition to any dinner party. It also makes a wonderfully delicious and beautiful birthday cake when covered in Basic Buttercream Frosting (page 124) made with coconut extract and toasted coconut flakes.

Makes: 8 to 10 servings

1 cup blanched almond flour

¼ cup coconut flour

½ teaspoon baking soda

¼ teaspoon salt

½ cup unsweetened coconut flakes

½ cup honey

½ cup (1 stick) unsalted butter, softened

3 large eggs, separated, room temperature

¼ cup Coconut Milk (page 130)

¼ cup SCD Yogurt (page 129)

1 teaspoon coconut extract

½ teaspoon pure vanilla extract

Preheat the oven to 350°F. Line a 9-inch round or square cake pan with parchment paper.

In a bowl, whisk together the flours, baking soda, salt, and coconut flakes, making sure there are no clumps. In a separate bowl, mix together the honey, butter, egg yolks, coconut milk, yogurt, and extracts. Whip the egg whites until soft peaks form. Add the butter mixture to the flour mixture, and stir to combine. Fold in the egg whites a third at a time until no white is visible. Pour the batter into the prepared cake pan.

Bake for 25 to 30 minutes, or until a cake tester inserted in the center comes out clean. Allow the cake to cool completely, at least 2 hours, before removing it from the pan. Store the cake covered in the refrigerator for up to one week.

Decorating the Cake

After the cake has cooled, you can frost it with the coconut buttercream frosting and gently press toasted coconut flakes into the frosting on the sides and sprinkle them on top.

White Cupcakes

Okay, okay, this can be made into cake, too, but cupcakes are just so much fun! Top them with frosting for a classic birthday treat. The flavor and texture are exactly like so-called normal cupcakes. Your friends and family will devour them—that is, if you don't eat them all first.

Makes: 12 servings

2 cups blanched almond flour

½ teaspoon baking soda

¼ teaspoon salt

½ cup (1 stick) unsalted butter, softened

½ cup dry curd cottage cheese (DCCC)

2 large eggs, room temperature

¼ cup SCD Yogurt (page 129)

1 teaspoon pure vanilla extract (page 132)

½ teaspoon pure almond extract (page 133)

Preheat the oven to 350°F. Place paper liners in a muffin tin.

In a bowl, combine the flour, baking soda, and salt. In a separate bowl, mix together the butter, DCCC, eggs, yogurt, and extracts. Add the butter mixture to the flour mixture, and stir to combine. Divide the batter evenly among the cupcake liners, filling no more than three-quarters full.

Bake for 25 to 30 minutes, or until a tester inserted in the center comes out clean. Allow the cupcakes to cool completely before frosting them. These can be stored covered in the refrigerator for up to one week.

Make It a Cake

You can make this into a cake instead of cupcakes by pouring the batter into a parchment paper–lined 9 inch cake pan. Bake for 35 to 40 minutes, or until a cake tester inserted in the middle comes out clean.

Jalapeño Cheddar Muffins

A little spicy and a little cheesy, these muffins are very similar to corn muffins. I like to serve them with a bowl of chili on a cold winter day.

Makes: 12 servings

1 cup blanched almond flour

½ cup coconut flour

½ teaspoon baking soda

½ teaspoon salt

3 large eggs, room temperature

1 cup Nut Milk (page 128) or Coconut Milk (page 130)

3 tablespoons unsalted butter, melted

2 tablespoons honey

1 teaspoon apple cider vinegar

1 jalapeño, diced

½ cup shredded cheddar cheese

Preheat the oven to 350°F. Place paper liners in a muffin tin.

In a bowl, whisk together the flours, baking soda, and salt, making sure there are no clumps. In a separate bowl, mix together the eggs, milk, butter, honey, and vinegar. Add the egg mixture to the flour mixture, and stir until fully combined. Fold in the jalapeño and the cheese. Divide the batter evenly among the muffin cups, filling each no more than three-quarters full.

Bake for 15 to 20 minutes, or until a tester inserted in the center of one muffin comes out clean. Enjoy hot or at room temperature. Store in airtight containers at room temperature for up to four days, or refrigerate for up to two weeks.

King Cake

This is a celebratory cake frequently made during Mardi Gras, but you can enjoy it any day of the year. A traditional king cake is made with yeast and has more of a bread-like texture. This version has the same flavor, although it is more like a sweet, spicy pound cake than bread. Cover it with Basic Buttercream Frosting (page 124), but make it a true king cake by adding color to the frosting with purple, green, and gold vegetable dyes.

Makes: 8 to 10 servings

3 cups blanched almond flour

½ teaspoon baking soda

½ teaspoon salt

1 cup (2 sticks) unsalted butter, room temperature

¼ cup honey

4 large eggs, separated, room temperature

1 teaspoon pure vanilla extract

1 teaspoon lemon zest

1 teaspoon ground cinnamon

¼ teaspoon ground nutmeg

Preheat the oven to 350°F. Line a 9-inch cake pan with parchment paper or spray the inside surface with oil.

In a bowl, whisk together the almond flour, baking soda, and salt. In a separate bowl, beat the butter and honey until it is light in color and it becomes very creamy. Add the egg yolks one at a time, mixing between additions. Add the vanilla, lemon zest, and spices. Add the butter mixture to the flour mixture, and stir until combined. In another bowl, whip the egg whites until soft peaks form. Fold the egg whites into the cake batter, incorporating a third of the whites at a time. It will be thick at first but will become lighter as the egg whites are incorporated. Pour the cake batter into the prepared pan.

Bake for 25 to 30 minutes, or until the edges begin to pull away from the pan and a cake tester inserted in the center comes out clean. Allow to cool completely before decorating. Store covered at room temperature for up to four days, or refrigerated for up to one week.

Lemon Yogurt Cake

Yogurt cakes are common in Europe, especially France. This version is quick and easy to throw together, which makes it a perfect last-minute dessert. It can be drizzled with a little honey or topped with fresh berries or Fruit Sauce (page 127). This recipe uses cashew butter for its light flavor and color. You can use another nut butter if you prefer its flavor, but it will result in a darker cake.

Makes: 8 to 10 servings

4 large eggs, separated, room temperature

¼ cup honey

¼ cup cashew butter

1 cup SCD Yogurt (page 129)

1 tablespoon lemon zest

½ cup fresh lemon juice (about 3 large lemons)

Preheat the oven to 350°F. Line a 9-inch cake pan with parchment paper or spray the inside surface with oil.

In a bowl, beat the egg yolks and honey until the mixture becomes much lighter in color. Add the cashew butter, yogurt, lemon zest, and lemon juice, and mix. Mix for another minute, until well combined. In a separate bowl, whip the egg whites until stiff peaks form. Gently fold the egg whites into the cake batter, incorporating a third of the whites at a time. Pour the batter into the prepared cake pan.

Bake for 30 to 40 minutes, or until a cake tester inserted into the center comes out clean. Allow the cake to cool before serving. Store covered in the refrigerator for up to one week.

Peach Muffins

This recipe really highlights the flavor of fresh peaches, although you can use frozen peaches when fresh ones are out of season. The muffin is not too sweet, and the peach flavor shines through.

Makes: 12 servings

1¾ cups blanched almond flour

1 teaspoon baking soda

½ teaspoon salt

½ cup SCD Yogurt (page 129)

¼ cup honey

1 large egg

1 teaspoon pure vanilla extract

1 cup peeled and diced peaches, fresh or frozen

Preheat the oven to 400°F. Place paper liners in a muffin tin.

In a bowl, combine the flour, baking soda, and salt. In a separate bowl, whisk together the yogurt, honey, egg, and vanilla. Add the yogurt mixture to the flour mixture, and lightly combine. Fold in the peaches. Divide the batter evenly among the 12 muffin cups.

Bake for 15 to 20 minutes, or until the muffins are golden and a tester inserted in the center of one comes out clean. Enjoy hot or room temperature. Store in airtight containers at room temperature for up to four days, or refrigerated for up to one week.

Peanut Butter Banana Muffins

This recipe is a tribute to Elvis Presley and his love of peanut butter, banana, and bacon sandwiches. I didn't include any bacon in this muffin recipe because it is so good and vegetarian-friendly without it. However, if you are feeling adventurous, feel free to add a few slices of cooked bacon to make it more like the Elvis sandwich. You can easily make these muffins into dessert by topping them with Banana Frosting (page 126).

Makes: 12 muffins

¾ cup pure, natural creamy peanut butter

2 ripe medium bananas

1 tablespoon honey

4 large eggs

½ teaspoon baking soda

Preheat the oven to 350°F. Place paper liners in a muffin tin.

In a bowl, combine the peanut butter, bananas, and honey. Add the eggs one at a time, mixing between additions. Add the baking soda, mixing until just combined. Divide the batter among the muffin cups until they are three-quarters full (about ¼ cup in each).

Bake for 12 to 15 minutes, or until a cake tester inserted in the center of a muffin comes out clean. Enjoy hot or room temperature. Store in airtight containers at room temperature for up to four days, or refrigerated for up to two weeks.

Peanut Butter Cake

This retro cake is moist and tender, thanks to the peanut butter and the SCD Yogurt. The cake isn't overwhelmingly sweet, so it makes a great base for these sweet toppings. Peanut butter and chocolate are a classic combination, so make sure to try this with Cocoa Butter Frosting (page 125). It is also delicious with Banana Frosting (page 126), or go a little crazy and use both.

Makes: 8 to 10 servings

1½ cups blanched almond flour

½ teaspoon baking soda

½ cup peanut butter

3 large eggs

⅓ cup SCD Yogurt (page 129)

¼ cup honey

¼ cup coconut oil

1 teaspoon pure vanilla extract

Preheat the oven to 350°F. Prepare a 9-inch cake pan by lining it with parchment or buttering the inside surface.

In a bowl, combine the flour and baking soda. In a separate bowl, mix together the peanut butter, eggs, yogurt, honey, oil, and vanilla. Add the peanut butter mixture to the flour mixture, and stir until completely blended. Pour the batter into the prepared cake pan.

Bake for 20 to 25 minutes, or until a cake tester inserted in the center comes out clean. Allow to cool completely before decorating. Store covered in the refrigerator for up to one week.

Almond Olive Oil Cake

Rustic and light, this cake is right for any occasion. You can even enjoy it for breakfast with a little fresh fruit or a drizzle of honey.

Makes: 8 to 10 servings

1 cup blanched almond flour

1 tablespoon coconut flour

½ cup honey

¼ teaspoon salt

4 large eggs, separated, room temperature

½ cup olive oil

3 tablespoons almond butter

1 teaspoon almond extract

Preheat the oven to 350°F. Prepare a 9-inch round cake pan by lining it with parchment paper and greasing the sides with oil.

In a bowl, mix together the flours, honey, salt, egg yolks, oil, almond butter, and almond extract. The batter will thicken as the coconut flour absorbs some of the liquid. In a separate bowl, beat the egg whites until soft peaks form. Fold the beaten whites into the batter, incorporating a third of the whites at a time, until there are no visible whites. Pour the batter into the prepared cake pan.

Bake for 30 to 40 minutes, or until the cake is lightly browned and a cake tester comes out clean. Allow to cool completely before removing from the pan. Store in airtight containers at room temperature for up to four days, or refrigerated for up to two weeks.

Classic Blueberry Muffins

These blueberry muffins are very similar to so called "normal" muffins made with all-purpose flour and they are likely to fool anyone not following SCD. Blueberry muffins are a great way to start any day. Once baked, they are an easy grab-and-go option in the morning.

Makes: 6 servings

1 cup blanched almond flour

¼ cup coconut flour

½ teaspoon baking soda

½ teaspoon salt

¼ cup coconut oil or unsalted butter, softened

2 large eggs, separated, room temperature

⅓ cup honey

¼ cup SCD Yogurt (page 129)

1 teaspoon lemon zest

1 teaspoon pure vanilla extract

1 cup fresh or frozen blueberries

Preheat the oven to 400°F. Place paper liners in a muffin tin.

In a bowl, whisk together the flours, baking soda, and salt, making sure there are no clumps. In a separate bowl, mix together the oil or butter, egg yolks, honey, yogurt, lemon zest, and vanilla until very well combined. In a clean bowl, whip the egg whites until soft peaks form. Add the oil or butter mixture to the flour mixture, and stir until combined. Fold the egg whites into the batter. Evenly distribute the batter among the muffin cups, filling each cup no more than three-quarters full. Divide the blueberries among the muffins, placing them on top. You can push them in slightly, but there is no need. They will sink slightly during baking.

Bake for 15 to 20 minutes, until the tops are golden brown and a cake tester inserted in the center of a muffin comes out clean. Enjoy hot or room temperature. Store in airtight containers at room temperature for up to four days, or refrigerated for up to two weeks.

Strawberry Shortcake

This is what summer is all about! The shortbread is soft and sweet, the strawberries add a saucy tang and topped with rich and decadent whipped coconut cream, this is quite an indulgent dessert. Bring this shortcake along on a picnic or to a barbecue for some fun build-your-own-dessert action. Shortcake is the perfect vehicle for strawberries, or any berries.

Makes: 8 servings

FOR THE SHORTCAKE

2 cups blanched almond flour

⅓ cup coconut flour

½ teaspoon baking soda

½ cup (1 stick) unsalted butter, softened

¼ cup honey

1 cup Coconut Cream (page 130)

1 large egg, room temperature

FOR THE FRUIT SAUCE

2 cups strawberries

2 tablespoons honey

FOR THE WHIPPED CREAM

1 cup Coconut Cream (page 130)

1 teaspoon honey

½ teaspoon pure vanilla extract

Preheat the oven to 350°F. Line a baking sheet with parchment paper.

Start by making the shortcake dough. In a bowl, whisk together the flours and the baking soda, making sure there are no clumps. In a separate bowl, mix together the butter, honey, coconut cream, and egg. Add the butter mixture to the flour mixture, and stir to combine. Divide the dough into eight portions, and roll each portion into a circle on the baking sheet, leaving about 1 inch between portions. Bake for 15 to 20 minutes, or until a tester inserted in the center of a shortcake comes out clean.

While the shortcake bakes, puree the strawberries. Place the strawberry puree and the honey in a small pan over medium heat. Heat until the sauce begins to simmer. Pour the sauce into a bowl, and refrigerate until ready to serve.

To make the whipped cream, place the coconut cream in a bowl and whip until soft peaks form. Add the honey and vanilla, and whip until combined. Serve immediately, or refrigerate until ready to use and rewhip into peaks.

To serve, cut the shortcakes in half. Spoon fruit sauce and whipped cream on the center of one half, and gently place the other half on top.

Zucchini Muffins

When summer's bounty of zucchini overflows, these muffins come to the rescue. They are slightly sweet, fluffy, and packed full of nutrients like vitamin C and folate. You can use fresh or frozen shredded zucchini, but make sure to squeeze out all of the excess water before mixing it into the batter.

Makes: 12 servings

2 cups almond flour

¼ cup coconut flour

1 teaspoon baking soda

1 teaspoon ground cinnamon

¼ teaspoon ground nutmeg

½ teaspoon salt

2 large eggs, separated

¼ cup coconut oil or unsalted butter, melted

½ cup honey

2 teaspoons pure vanilla extract

2 cups shredded zucchini

Preheat the oven to 350°F. Line a muffin tin with paper liners.

In a bowl, whisk together the flours, baking soda, spices, and salt, making sure there are no clumps in the mix. In another bowl, mix together the egg yolks, oil or butter, honey, and vanilla. In a clean bowl, whip the egg whites until soft peaks form. Add the honey mixture and the zucchini to the flour mixture, combining thoroughly. Fold the beaten whites into the batter, until there are no visible whites. Fill each muffin cup with batter until three-quarters full. Bake for 20 to 30 minutes, or until the tops are golden brown and a tester inserted into a muffin comes out clean. Enjoy hot or room temperature. Store in airtight containers at room temperature for up to four days, or refrigerated for up to two weeks.

Pineapple Upside-Down Cake

This is definitely a dessert that you'll want for your next get-together. It is so wonderfully yummy and pretty to serve. The date paste works well as a substitute for the brown sugar syrup typically used, and the parchment paper helps the cake release easily from the pan. Most of the flavor comes from the pineapple, so be sure to choose a sweet one.

Makes: 10 to 12 servings

¼ cup Date Paste (page 131)

½ fresh pineapple, peeled, cored, and cut into ½ inch slices

1½ cups blanched almond flour

½ teaspoon baking soda

¼ cup honey

¼ cup (½ stick) unsalted butter, softened

¼ cup Coconut Milk (page 130) or Nut Milk (page 128)

1 large egg, room temperature

Preheat the oven to 350°F. Line a 9-inch round or square cake pan with parchment paper, and butter the sides.

Spread the date paste evenly on the bottom of the pan. Arrange the pineapple slices on top of the date paste. In a bowl, mix together the flour and baking soda. Add the honey, butter, milk, and egg, stirring until well combined. Pour the batter over the pineapple slices in the pan, and spread until even.

Bake for 25 to 30 minutes, or until a cake tester inserted in the center comes out clean. Remove the pan from the oven and allow the cake to cool slightly, about 10 to 15 minutes, then place a serving plate face-down over the cake. Carefully, pressing the pan into the plate, flip the cake over. The cake should come out of the pan onto the plate, but tap the pan gently if the cake needs some help. Serve warm.

Store any remaining cake covered in the refrigerator for up to a week.

TIP: A pineapple is ripe when a center leaf from the top pulls out easily.

Berry DCCC Cake

On the outside, this cake appears to be like any other cake, but slice into it and you'll find juicy berries hiding on the bottom. DCCC stands for "dry curd cottage cheese." It is very similar to ricotta, but unlike ricotta is SCD legal. You can determine the sweetness of your cake by adjusting the honey in this recipe, which is why a range is listed.

Makes: 10 to 12 servings

2 cups blanched almond flour

½ teaspoon baking soda

¼ teaspoon salt

½ cup (1 stick) unsalted butter, softened

3 large eggs, room temperature

½ cup dry curd cottage cheese (DCCC)

¼ to ⅓ cup honey

¼ cup Nut Milk (page 128) or Coconut Milk (page 130)

2 teaspoons pure vanilla extract

½ teaspoon orange zest

2 cups fresh or frozen berries

Preheat the oven to 350°F. Line a 9-inch round or square cake pan with parchment paper, and butter the sides.

In a bowl, combine the flour, baking soda, and salt. In a separate bowl, mix together the butter, eggs, DCCC, honey, milk, vanilla, and orange zest. Add the butter mixture to the flour mixture, and stir to combine. Arrange the berries in a single layer in the cake pan. Pour the batter over the berries, and spread until even.

Bake for 30 to 40 minutes, or until a cake tester inserted in the center comes out clean. Allow the cake to cool completely before removing it from the pan. Store covered in the refrigerator for up to one week.

Strawberry Scones

This is sweet and delicate, falling somewhere between a biscuit and cake. It is simply wonderful! Top with a little Coconut Cream (page 130) and a bit of honey (the SCD version of Devonshire cream). Another great aspect of this scone? You can use other fruits in the same proportion as the strawberries. For a little variety, try this recipe with other berries, peaches, or even mango.

Makes: 8 scones

1 cup blanched almond flour

½ cup coconut flour

1 teaspoon baking soda

½ cup (1 stick) unsalted butter, softened

¼ cup honey

1 large egg, room temperature

¼ cup SCD Yogurt (page 129)

1 cup diced fresh strawberries

Preheat the oven to 350°F. Line a baking sheet with parchment paper.

In a bowl, whisk together the flours and baking soda. In a separate bowl, mix together the butter, honey, and egg. Stir the butter mixture into the flour mixture until completely incorporated. Fold in the yogurt and the strawberries. Form the dough into a ball, and flatten it until about 9 inches in diameter. Cut the dough four times across, until there are eight equal pieces. Arrange the pieces on the prepared baking sheet, leaving about 1 inch between pieces.

Bake for 25 to 30 minutes, or until lightly browned. Enjoy warm or at room temperature. Store any leftover scones in an airtight container for up to one week in the refrigerator.

Chapter 3
Cookies and Bars

Cinnamon Cookies

These cinnamon cookies were inspired by Biscoff cookies. The great part about these cookies is that they use date paste as a sweetener instead of sugar.

Makes: 24 cookies

3 tablespoons coconut flour

½ teaspoon baking soda

¼ cup Date Paste (page 131)

½ teaspoon ground cinnamon

¼ cup water

2 tablespoons coconut oil

Preheat the oven to 350°F. Line two baking sheets with parchment paper.

In a bowl, mix together all of the ingredients. Drop cookie batter by the tablespoon onto the baking sheets, leaving about 2 inches between cookies.

Bake for 10 to 15 minutes, or until the edges of the cookies are brown. If you like crunchier cookies, bake for an additional 2 to 3 minutes. Allow the cookies to cool on the cookie sheet before removing them. These can be stored in an airtight container at room temperature for up to a week or frozen for up to three months.

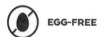 **EGG-FREE**

DCCC Thumbprint Cookies

This delightful little cookie is a colorful addition to a dessert tray. The addition of dry curd cottage cheese makes the cookie super light and crisp.

Makes: 24 cookies

1 cup blanched almond flour

¼ cup (½ stick) unsalted butter, cut into cubes

2 tablespoons dry curd cottage cheese (DCCC)

1 tablespoon honey

¼ cup SCD-friendly fruit jam*

*SCD-friendly jam is made with honey and is free of pectin. They may contain a small amount of gelatin to help the fruit set up, in place of pectin.

Preheat the oven to 350°F. Line two baking sheets with parchment paper.

In a bowl, mix together the flour, butter, DCCC, and honey. Spoon tablespoon-size circles of dough onto the parchment paper, leaving about 1½ inches between cookies to allow them to spread. Form a small divot in the center of each cookie, and fill it with the fruit jam.

Bake for 10 to 12 minutes, or until the edges begin to brown. Allow the cookies to cool on the baking sheet. Store at room temperature in an airtight container for up to one week or frozen for up to three months.

 EGG-FREE

Fruit and Nut Cookies

These sweet, crisp cookies will please even people who aren't following SCD, but I wouldn't blame you if you didn't want to share. Try adding assorted nuts and dried fruits for a diversity of flavors.

Makes: 20 cookies

1 cup blanched almond flour

¼ cup chopped nuts

¼ cup chopped dried, unsweetened fruit

¼ cup honey

1 teaspoon ground cinnamon

¼ teaspoon ground nutmeg

Preheat the oven to 350°F. Line two cookie sheets with parchment paper or spray them with oil. In a bowl, thoroughly mix together all of the ingredients. Evenly divide the batter into 20 portions, rolling each portion into a ball. Place them on the cookie sheets, leaving about 2 inches between cookies to allow them to spread.

Bake for 10 to 15 minutes, or until the edges are golden. Allow the cookies to cool completely on the baking sheet before serving. Store the cookies in an airtight container at room temperature for up to one week or in the freezer for up to three months.

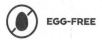 **EGG-FREE**

Cashew Cake Cookies

These are perfect for the times when you can't decide whether to have a cookie or cake. Why not have both? These cookies are a bit like muffin tops without their bottoms. This is a very basic recipe that you can jazz up with the addition of dried fruit, seeds, or other types of nuts.

Makes: 18 to 22 cookies

2 cups cashew butter

1 large egg, room temperature

½ cup Date Paste (page 131)

¼ cup honey

½ teaspoon baking soda

¼ teaspoon salt

½ cup chopped cashews

Preheat the oven to 350°F. Line two baking sheets with parchment paper.

In a bowl, thoroughly combine all of the ingredients. Drop balls of dough by the tablespoon onto the baking sheet, leaving about 1 inch between cookies to allow them to spread. Bake for 10 to 14 minutes, or until the edges have browned. Allow the cookies to cool slightly before serving.

TIP: You can use other types of nut butters, in place of cashew butter, for a different flavor.

Brown Butter Sage Cookies

The sweet, nutty flavor of brown butter complements savory sage. These cookies can be made sweeter or more savory simply by adjusting the amount of salt and honey added to the batter. Including sage in the cookies creates beautiful flecks of green throughout.

Makes: 18 to 20 cookies

⅓ cup (⅔ stick) unsalted butter

¼ cup sage leaves

1 cup blanched almond flour

¼ cup coconut flour

½ teaspoon baking soda

¼ teaspoon salt plus ¼ teaspoon if making a savory cookie

1 large egg, room temperature

¼ cup honey if making a sweet cookie

Preheat the oven to 350°F. Line two baking sheets with parchment paper.

In a small pot, warm the butter over medium-low heat. After about 10 minutes, white fat solids will rise to the top. With a spoon, carefully remove the solids. Place the sage leaves in the hot butter, and cook until the edges curl and the leaves turn dark green. Remove the sage, and place on a paper towel to cool. Continue to cook the butter until it turns light brown, about 10 to 20 minutes.

While the butter is cooking, mix together the flours, baking soda, ¼ teaspoon of salt (and an additional ¼ teaspoon if making a savory cookie), and egg in a bowl. Add the honey if making a sweet cookie. Stir in the brown butter. Crumble up the sage, and mix into the dough.

Form walnut-sized balls of dough, and place on the baking sheets, leaving about 2 inches between balls. Gently press the balls down until they are about 2 inches in diameter. Bake for 10 to 12 minutes, or until the edges are browned.

Homemade Energy Bars

These are similar to the fruit and nut bars Lara Bars, and are incredibly easy to make. While this isn't actually a baking recipe, it is a very popular snack that everyone could benefit from knowing how to make, since they are so delicious. These make a great on-the-go snack.

Makes: 4 to 6 bars

1 cup cashews, toasted   ½ cup Date Paste (page 131)

In a food processor, pulse the cashews until they are about the size of pebbles. Add the date paste, and pulse until they are combined. Divide the mixture into four or six portions, and place each on a 6-inch-square piece of wax paper or parchment paper. Form each portion into a square or rectangle, and fold the paper over the top. Place the bars in an airtight container, and store in the refrigerator for up to one month until ready to eat.

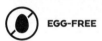 **EGG-FREE**

Variations

APPLE CINNAMON ENERGY BAR: Add ¼ cup chopped dried apples and ¼ teaspoon cinnamon.

COCONUT ENERGY BAR: Add ¼ cup coconut flakes and 1 tablespoon coconut oil.

To create your own variety, add up to ¼ cup of other ingredients and up to 1½ teaspoons of spices.

Almond Vanilla Granola

Simple to make, this granola is yummy with a little nut milk or in a fruit and yogurt parfait. It is so much more affordable to make your own grain-free granola than to purchase it from the store. It is easy to switch up the flavors with a few additional ingredients.

Makes: About 4 cups

1 cup raw sunflower seeds

1 cup raw almonds

1 cup raw pumpkin seeds

¼ cup honey

1 tablespoon olive oil or melted coconut oil

1 teaspoon pure vanilla extract

½ teaspoon ground cinnamon

¼ teaspoon salt

½ cup dried, unsweetened fruit, such as apples or raisins

Preheat the oven to 325°F. Line a baking sheet with parchment paper.

In a food processor, pulse the sunflower seeds to a medium grind. Add the almonds and pumpkin seeds, and pulse until just broken up into smaller pieces. Pulse for longer if you want a very fine-textured granola. Place the processed seeds and nuts in a bowl, and add the honey, oil, vanilla, cinnamon, and salt. Mix thoroughly. Spread it out evenly on the parchment paper.

Bake for about 40 minutes, stirring every 8 minutes to avoid burning. Pay special attention to the edges. Once all of the mixture is evenly browned, remove the baking sheet from the oven. Using a spatula, mix the dried fruit into the hot granola. Allow to cool for 10 to 15 minutes. Once cooled, break up the granola and store in an airtight container.

 EGG-FREE

Variations

TROPICAL: Add flaked coconut, chopped macadamia nuts, and chopped dried pineapple.

APPLE CINNAMON: Use both chopped dried apple and raisins, and increase the cinnamon to 1 teaspoon.

PECAN PIE: Use pecans in place of almonds, and choose chopped dates for the dried fruit.

Honey Lavender Shortbread Cookies

This is a posh little treat to whip up for teatime. Sweet and floral, these flavorful cookies are unique, and beautiful with little specks of lavender. You can use rosemary instead of lavender if you want to switch it up.

Makes: 24 cookies

1 cup coconut flour

½ cup (1 stick) butter or coconut oil

½ cup honey

½ teaspoon dried lavender

Preheat the oven to 350°F. Line a baking sheet with parchment paper.

In a large bowl, mix together all of the ingredients. Scoop tablespoon-size portions of the dough, roll them into balls, and place them on the baking sheet, leaving 1 inch in between each cookie. Flatten them with your hand until about ½-inch thick.

Bake for 8 to 10 minutes, or until the edges begin to brown. Cool on a wire rack. Once cooled, store the cookies in an airtight container for up to one week at room temperature and up to three months in the freezer.

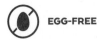 EGG-FREE

Cherry Nut Bars

This bar is incredibly easy to make and great for a snack when you are on the go. The recipe is very flexible: You can substitute your favorite nuts, seeds, and fruits in the same proportions and still have a delicious but healthy energy bar.

Makes: 8 bars

1 cup raw pecans

1 cup raw pistachios

1 cup raw almonds

1 cup dried, unsweetened cherries

4 dates, pits removed

¼ cup honey

¼ teaspoon salt

Preheat the oven to 300°F. Lightly oil a 9-inch square pan.

In a food processor, combine the nuts. Process for about 10 to 15 seconds, or until the nuts are about a quarter of the size they were. Add the remaining ingredients, and continue to process until everything is combined, about 10 seconds. Pour the nut mixture into the prepared pan. Spread evenly, pressing down to flatten the mixture.

Bake for 15 to 20 minutes, or until the nuts become very fragrant and are lightly browned. Allow to cool completely before cutting into bars. To portion, cut in half, then cut across into four equal bars. To store, separate each bar with parchment paper and store in an airtight container at room temperature for up to one week or in the freezer for up to three months.

 EGG-FREE

TIP: Watch the nut mixture carefully when it is in the oven. Nuts and honey can burn easily.

Spice Cookies

Wonderful for the holidays, these cookies remind me of the ones my grandma makes every year as gifts. You can frost them with Buttercream Frosting (page 124) or enjoy them as they are. The date paste acts like molasses in this recipe, giving the rich flavor and dark color that you expect.

Makes: 24 cookies

1 cup blanched almond flour

¼ cup coconut flour

1 teaspoon baking soda

1½ teaspoon ground cinnamon

1½ teaspoon ground ginger

½ teaspoon ground cloves

¼ teaspoon ground allspice

¼ teaspoon salt

¾ cup (1½ sticks) unsalted butter

¼ cup Date Paste (page 131)

¼ cup honey

1 large egg, room temperature

1 teaspoon pure vanilla extract

In a bowl, combine the flours, baking soda, spices, and salt. Use a whisk to stir, as coconut flour can sometimes clump. In a separate bowl, beat together the butter, date paste, and honey to combine, then add the egg and vanilla. Add the flour mixture to the butter mixture, and mix until combined. Refrigerate the dough for 2 hours, or up to three days.

To bake, preheat the oven to 350°F. Divide the dough into 24 even portions, and roll them into balls. They should be about 1 inch in diameter. Place them on a lined baking sheet, 2 inches apart. Bake for 10 to 18 minutes, or until the edges are very brown. Allow the cookies to cool on the baking sheet for about 5 minutes before removing them.

Meringue Cookies

Crisp and sweet, these cookies make a good crunchy treat. You can vary the size and use them to decorate cakes and other cookies with a little frosting. You can also place a little custard or jam between two cookies for a meringue sandwich. Since honey is the sweetener, these cookies are golden instead of snowy white like meringues made with sugar.

Makes: 3 dozen cookies

¼ cup honey

6 large egg whites, chilled

1 teaspoon fresh lemon juice or white vinegar

1 teaspoon pure vanilla extract

Preheat the oven to 200°F. Line two baking sheets with parchment paper.

In a pot over medium-high heat, heat the honey until it boils, and allow it to boil for about 3 minutes, or until the temperature reaches 235 degrees. Use a candy thermometer to check the temperature. In a bowl, whip the egg whites and lemon juice until stiff peaks form. While continuing to whisk, slowly drizzle the hot honey into the egg whites and the vanilla, whisking until incorporated. The mixture will become smooth and glossy.

Using a piping bag or a spoon, create mounds, stars, nests, or any shape you like of meringues, leaving about 1 inch between cookies.

Bake for 1 to 2 hours, until the meringues are lightly browned. Allow the meringues to cool completely on the baking sheet before removing them. Store at room temperature in an airtight container. These are best the same day, but can be stored for up to one week.

TIP: These cookies are sticky due to the honey and should be stored without touching each other.

Vanilla Cookies

A simple cookie that serves as a base for frostings or jam, or can be served with coffee, is essential. This one is easy and takes only about 20 minutes to make, from start to finish.

Makes: 20 cookies

1 cup blanched almond flour

1 tablespoon coconut flour

1 teaspoon baking soda

½ cup (1 stick) unsalted butter or coconut oil

¼ cup honey

1 large egg, room temperature

1 tablespoon pure vanilla extract

Preheat the oven to 325°F. Line a cookie sheet with parchment paper or spray it with oil.

In a bowl, whisk together the flours and the baking soda. In a separate bowl, mix together the butter or oil, honey, egg, and vanilla. Add the flour mixture to the honey mixture, and stir until completely combined. Drop the batter by tablespoon onto the cookie sheet, leaving 2 inches between cookies.

Bake for 10 to 15 minutes, or until the edges start to brown. Once cooled, store the cookies in an airtight container for up to two weeks at room temperature or three months in the freezer.

Coconut Macaroons

This simple recipe has only five ingredients, but the cookies are anything but simple. What look like fluffy, white pillows of coconut are actually dense, chewy cookies. These cute little cookies always make it onto my Christmas cookie gift plate, but they are delicious any time of year.

Makes: About 2 dozen cookies

4 large egg whites, room temperature

½ cup honey

1 teaspoon pure vanilla extract

¼ teaspoon salt

4 cups finely grated, unsweetened coconut flakes

Preheat the oven to 300°F. Line two baking sheets with parchment paper.

Whip the egg whites until soft peaks form. Meanwhile, in a small pan over medium-high heat, heat the honey until it boils. With the mixer running, slowly add the hot honey to the egg whites, then add the vanilla and salt, whisking until the ingredients are incorporated. Fold in the coconut flakes. The mixture will be thick. Drop by the spoonful onto the baking sheets, leaving about 1 inch between cookies.

Bake for 15 to 20 minutes, or until the edges begin to brown. The cookies will be very soft when they come out of the oven but will firm up as they cool. Allow them to cool for about 10 minutes before serving. Stored in an airtight container, the cookies will keep for up to three days at room temperature or up to one week in the refrigerator.

Peanut Butter Cookies

A childhood favorite, peanut butter is a good source of niacin and vitamin E. This recipe is simple and quick to make, and it's a fun baking project that you can do with kids. The cookies can be soft or crisp, depending on how long you bake them.

Makes: About 24 cookies

1 cup peanut butter

⅓ cup Date Paste (page 131)

¼ cup (½ stick) unsalted butter, softened

1 large egg, room temperature

½ teaspoon baking soda

½ teaspoon pure vanilla extract

¼ teaspoon salt

Preheat the oven to 350°F. Line a baking sheet with parchment paper.

Mix together all of the ingredients. Using a tablespoon, scoop the dough out and roll it between your hands to form into balls, and place on the baking sheet 1½ inches apart. Gently press a fork into the top of each cookie, forming a crisscross.

Bake for about 10 minutes for soft cookies and about 15 minutes for crisper cookies. The edges should be brown. For even crisper cookies, add an additional 3 to 5 minutes. Allow the cookies to cool completely before removing them from the baking sheet. Once cooled, store the cookies in an airtight container for up to two weeks at room temperature or three months in the freezer.

"Oatmeal" Raisin Cookies

The sweet smell of cinnamon floats out of your oven while these cookies bake. Instead of rolled oats, this recipe uses coconut flakes and almond meal for texture. These cookies are egg-free but still fluffy, thanks to date paste.

Makes: 15 to 18 cookies

1 cup almond butter

¼ cup Date Paste (page 131)

¼ cup (½ stick) unsalted butter, softened

1 tablespoon honey

1 tablespoon coconut flour

½ teaspoon baking soda

½ teaspoon ground cinnamon

⅛ teaspoon salt

¼ cup raisins

2 tablespoons finely grated, unsweetened coconut

1 tablespoon almond meal

Preheat the oven to 350°F. Line two baking sheets with parchment paper. Mix together the almond butter, date paste, butter, honey, coconut flour, baking soda, cinnamon, and salt. Once the ingredients are well combined, add the raisins, coconut flakes, and almond meal, stirring until evenly incorporated. Drop the dough onto the baking sheets, a tablespoon at a time, leaving 2 inches between cookies.

Bake for 12 to 15 minutes or until the edges begin to brown. Allow the cookies to cool completely before removing them from the baking sheet. Once cooled, store the cookies separated by parchment in an airtight container for up to two weeks at room temperature or three months in the freezer.

 EGG-FREE

Vanilla Shortbread Cookies

Nut-free and egg-free, these light, crisp cookies make a tasty, quick treat. They are everything you want from shortbread. This is a very basic version of a shortbread cookie recipe, so feel free to change the extract to add some variety.

Makes: 24 cookies

¾ cup coconut flour

½ cup (1 stick) butter or coconut oil

¼ cup honey

1 tablespoon pure vanilla extract

Preheat the oven to 350°F. Line a baking sheet with parchment paper.

Mix together all of the ingredients. Using a tablespoon, scoop the dough and roll the dough into balls, and place them on the baking sheet, leaving about 1 inch between each cookie. Flatten them with your hand until they are about ½ inch thick. Bake for 8 to 10 minutes, or until the edges begin to brown. Once cooled, store the cookies in an airtight container for up to two weeks at room temperature or three months in the freezer.

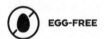 **EGG-FREE**

Black Bean "Brownies"

Missing chocolate? While this isn't exactly a chocolate brownie, it is similar. The combination of coffee and cocoa butter tastes surprisingly chocolaty. The black beans give these "brownies" their very fudgy texture as well as giving you a dose of extra fiber. If you prefer something a little more cakelike, try the Black Bean "Chocolate" Cake on page 44. Make sure that you prepare your black beans according to the SCD guidelines, by soaking them overnight before cooking them.

Makes: 16 brownies

¾ cups cooked black beans*

2 large eggs, room temperature

½ cup cocoa butter, melted

2 tablespoons honey

⅓ cup Date Paste (page 131)

¼ cup espresso or strong brewed coffee or 2 teaspoons coffee extract

½ teaspoon pure vanilla extract

¼ teaspoon salt

*Beans should be soaked in water overnight and then rinsed before cooking them. Boil for about 15 minutes and then simmer for about 35 minutes, or until the beans are soft. Be sure to remove any scum that rises to the top.

Preheat the oven to 350°F. Butter a 9 × 9-inch square cake pan or line it with parchment paper.

In a blender, combine all of the ingredients, pulsing until everything is very smooth. Pour the batter into the prepared pan.

Bake for 40 to 45 minutes. The batter will still be a little gooey, but it will become firmer as it cools. Allow to cool completely before serving. Once cooled, store the brownies covered for up to three days at room temperature, two weeks in the fridge, or three months in the freezer.

Cocoa Butter Blondie

Rich and fudgy, this blondie is a perfect treat to satisfy your sugar cravings. It smells heavenly while baking and tastes yummy when still a little warm from the oven.

Makes: 12 blondies

4 large eggs, room temperature

½ cup Date Paste (page 131)

¼ cup honey

1 teaspoon pure vanilla extract

¼ teaspoon salt

1 cup cocoa butter, melted

1 cup blanched almond flour

Preheat the oven to 325°F. Prepare a square 9-inch square cake pan by lining it with parchment or buttering the inside surface.

In a bowl, mix together all of the ingredients. The batter will be pretty thin. Pour it into the prepared pan.

Bake for 20 to 25 minutes, until the edges begin to brown and the center of the cake is firm. The blondie will rise during baking but will settle during cooling. Allow to cool completely before serving. Once cooled, store the blondies covered for up to three days at room temperature, one month in the fridge, or three months in the freezer.

Lemon Bars

Buttery shortbread and tangy lemon curd combine to make this refreshing treat. You can easily adjust the tartness of the lemon by adding or subtracting the amount of zest. I love these lemon bars because they travel well and are easy to share or bring to a picnic.

Makes: 9 to 12 servings

FOR THE SHORTBREAD

½ cup coconut flour

½ cup (1 stick) unsalted butter, softened

2 large egg whites

2 tablespoons Date Paste (page 131)

¼ teaspoon salt

FOR THE FILLING

7 large egg yolks plus 2 large eggs, room temperature

1 cup honey

⅔ cup fresh lemon juice (about 3 lemons)

1 to 3 tablespoons lemon zest

½ teaspoon salt

1 tablespoon unsalted butter

Preheat the oven to 350°F. Line a 9-inch square cake pan with parchment paper and spray it with oil.

To make the shortbread, mix the ingredients until well combined. Press the dough into the bottom of the cake pan. Bake for 15 to 20 minutes, or until golden.

While the shortbread is cooling, make the filling. Mix together the egg yolks and whole eggs, honey, lemon juice, lemon zest, and salt in a pot. Place over medium-low heat, and stir until the filling begins to thicken. Pour through a fine-mesh strainer into a bowl. Stir in the butter until it melts. Pour the filling into the prepared cake pan.

Bake for 15 to 20 minutes. The lemon curd should start to set around the edges, and the center should be a little wobbly. Allow to cool for 30 to 45 minutes before cutting into bars. Once cooled, store the bars, covered, for up to two weeks in the fridge or three months in the freezer.

Chapter 4
Pies, Cobblers, and Crisps

Apple Pie

At my house, the holiday season always involves apple pie. I like to eat it when it is still warm, but it is equally delicious cooled. Leftovers become breakfast the next day. The secret to a crisp crust is to parbake it and to completely cook the filling on the stove before adding it to the crust. Use a variety of apples for the best flavor and texture. My favorite combinations include Granny Smith, Cortland, and Honeycrisp apples.

Makes: 6 to 8 servings

2 Pie Crusts (page 110)

4 large apples, peeled, cored, and sliced

¼ cup Date Paste (page 131)

½ teaspoon ground cinnamon

⅛ teaspoon ground nutmeg

⅛ teaspoon ground cloves

1 tablespoon fresh lemon juice

1 egg, beaten

Preheat the oven to 350°F. Prepare the pie crust dough, doubling the recipe on page 110. Divide the dough in half. Parbake the bottom pie crust for 10 to 15 minutes. Roll out the top crust, and refrigerate it while preparing the filling.

In a pot over medium-low heat, simmer the apples and lemon juice until softened, about 25 to 30 minutes, depending on the apples used. Stir in the date paste and spices. Spoon the apple mixture into the bottom crust. Remove the top crust from the refrigerator. Place the rolled-out dough over the filling, crimp the edges, and cut three ventilation slits on top. As an alternative, you can cut out designs with a knife or a cookie cutter and arrange them on top of the filling. Brush the beaten egg on the top crust or cutouts.

Bake for 20 to 30 minutes, or until the crust is golden brown. Allow the pie to cool slightly before serving. Once cooled, the pie can be wrapped and kept in the refrigerator for up to one week.

Cherry Pie

Whether sweet or sour, cherries make some of the best desserts. This recipe uses sweet cherries, but you can substitute sour cherries if you double the amount of date paste. The key to getting the right texture is to partially bake the bottom crust and to cook the cherry filling on the stove. This also lets you adjust the flavor of the filling until it is just right.

Makes: 6 to 8 servings

2 Pie Crusts (page 110)

5 cups fresh or frozen sweet cherries

¼ cup Date Paste (page 131)

1 tablespoon fresh lemon juice

1 tablespoon unsalted butter

1 large egg, beaten

Preheat the oven to 350°F. Prepare the pie crust dough, doubling the recipe on page 110. Divide the dough in half. Roll out and refrigerate the dough for the bottom crust. Parbake the bottom pie crust for 10 to 15 minutes. Roll out the top crust, and refrigerate it while preparing the filling.

In a pot over medium-low heat, stir the cherries and date paste together and simmer until they are very soft and the juices reduce by half, about 20 minutes. Stir in the lemon juice and butter, allowing the butter to melt completely. Pour the filling into the bottom crust. Remove the top crust from the refrigerator, and cut it into ribbons for a lattice top or cut out shapes to decorate the top of the pie. Weave the lattice top over the filling or place the cutouts on top. Brush the beaten egg on top of the lattice or cutouts.

Bake for 20 minutes, or until the lattice or cutouts are golden and crisp. Cool slightly before serving or cool completely. The pie can be wrapped and kept in the refrigerator for up to one week.

Fruit Tart

This stylish dessert is easy to dress up and sure to impress. You can use whatever soft fruits you like, such as fresh berries, plums, and peaches, or tropical choices like mango and kiwi. Any combination will be stunning. A small amount of fruit gelatin brushed over the top adds sheen to the fruit.

Makes: 6 to 8 servings

FOR THE CRUST
½ cup coconut flour

½ cup blanched almond flour

¼ cup (½ stick) unsalted butter

1 large egg, room temperature

1 tablespoon honey

FOR THE FILLING
2 cups Coconut Milk or Coconut Cream (page 130)

4 egg yolks

2 tablespoons honey

2 teaspoons gelatin powder

1 teaspoon pure vanilla extract

FOR THE GLAZE
½ cup fruit juice, such as apple, peach, or apricot

1 teaspoon gelatin powder

Preheat the oven to 350°F.

To make the crust, combine all of the ingredients in a food processor. Process until well combined. Alternatively, you can use your fingers to rub the flours and butter together until combined, then stir in the egg and honey. Press the dough into a tart shell or pie dish until the bottom and sides are evenly covered. Bake for 10 to 15 minutes, until golden.

To make the filling, whisk together the coconut milk or coconut cream, egg yolks, honey, and gelatin in a pot. Let sit for 5 minutes to allow the gelatin to bloom. Over medium-low heat, warm the mixture, stirring constantly. It will begin to thicken slightly and should coat a spoon. Do not let it come to a boil, as the egg yolks will curdle. Remove from the heat, and stir in the vanilla. Gently pour into the baked crust. Cover with plastic wrap, and let chill in the refrigerator. After at least 8 hours, arrange the berries or sliced fruit over the custard filling.

To make the glaze, pour the fruit juice into a small pot. Sprinkle the gelatin over the juice, and let sit for 5 minutes. Gently heat the juice over low heat, stirring occasionally, until the gelatin is completely dissolved. Allow to cool to room temperature. Using a pastry brush, brush the glaze over the top of the fruit. Allow the tart to cool in the refrigerator for at least 1 hour before serving. This is best eaten the same day, as the crust will become soggy over time.

Chicken Pot Pie

A meal that has been made for many centuries must be doing something right. An entire meal in one dish, pot pie is the ultimate comfort food. It is a tasty way to incorporate nutritious bone broth into more meals, if you have some on hand. Feel free to use other meats in the filling and to substitute beef or vegetable stock or bone broth.

Makes: 6 to 8 servings

1 Savory Pie Crust (page 111)

1 tablespoon unsalted butter or vegetable oil

1 medium yellow onion, diced

3 large celery stalks, diced

3 medium carrots, peeled and diced

1 cup diced vegetables, such as butternut squash, green beans, peas, or mushrooms (optional)

½ cup dry white wine

2 cups chicken stock or bone broth

½ cup Coconut Milk or Nut Milk (page 128)

½ teaspoon dried thyme or 1½ teaspoons fresh thyme

3 cups cooked and shredded chicken breasts (about 3 breasts)

salt and black pepper

Preheat the oven to 350°F. Following the directions on page 111, prepare the savory pie crust dough. Roll out the dough between two sheets of parchment paper or plastic wrap. Place on a flat surface, such as a cutting board, and chill in the refrigerator for 30 minutes.

In a medium pot over medium heat, melt the butter or oil. Add the onion, and cook until translucent, about 3 to 5 minutes, stirring occasionally. Add the celery, carrots, and other vegetables, if using. Cook for about 5 minutes, stirring occasionally. Then add the wine, and allow to simmer for about 2 minutes. Add the stock or bone broth, milk, and thyme, and continue to simmer. After a few minutes, add the shredded chicken, and season to taste with salt and pepper. Pour the mixture into a 9 × 13-inch baking dish.

Remove the pie crust from the refrigerator, and take off the top sheet of parchment paper or plastic wrap. Carefully lay the dough over the baking dish, covering it edge to edge, while pulling off the remaining sheet. Cut a couple of ventilation slits in the dough. Bake for 30 to 40 minutes, or until the crust is browned. Serve hot. The pie can be wrapped and kept in the refrigerator for up to one week.

TIP: Place foil in the bottom of your oven or place the baking dish onto a sheet pan. This makes for much easier cleanup if any liquid bubbles over the edges.

Banana Cream Pie

A favorite dessert of the 1950s, cream pie is deliciously retro. Typically, you would use all-purpose flour or cornstarch to thicken the filling, but since that is not an option in SCD baking, use gelatin instead. Give yourself plenty of time to make this pie, as it needs to set in the refrigerator for at least 8 hours.

Makes: 6 to 8 servings

1 Pie Crust (page 110)

2 cups Coconut Cream (page 130)

¼ cup honey

2 large eggs, room temperature

1½ teaspoons gelatin powder

½ teaspoon salt

2 medium ripe bananas, sliced

1 teaspoon pure vanilla extract

Preheat the oven to 350°F. Prepare the pie crust dough, and roll it out and refrigerate it as described on page 110. Bake the crust for 20 to 25 minutes, until golden brown. Allow to cool.

In a pot, whisk together the coconut cream, honey, eggs, gelatin, and salt. Let stand for 5 minutes, to give the gelatin time to bloom. Meanwhile, line the bottom of the cooled pie crust with the sliced bananas.

Heat the cream mixture over medium-low heat, stirring constantly. The mixture will begin to thicken slightly and should coat a spoon. Do not let it come to a boil, as the eggs will curdle. Remove from the heat, and stir in the vanilla. Gently pour the filling through a fine mesh strainer over the bananas in the pie crust.

Cover with plastic wrap, gently pressing the plastic wrap onto the surface of the filling. Place in the refrigerator, and allow to chill for at least 8 hours before serving. The pie can be wrapped and kept in the refrigerator for up to one week.

Onion Tart

A bit sweet and a bit savory, this tart is delicious served with a salad. It's a decadent vegetarian meal, or it can be made into mini tartlets for lovely hors d'oeuvres.

Makes: 6 to 8 servings or 24 mini tartlets

FOR THE CRUST

½ cup blanched almond flour

½ cup coconut flour

¼ cup (½ stick) unsalted butter, chilled and cut into cubes

1 large egg, room temperature

½ teaspoon salt

FOR THE FILLING

2 large sweet onions

1 pound dry curd cottage cheese (DCCC)

½ cup shredded cheese, such as Swiss or Gruyère

1 large egg, room temperature

¼ teaspoon salt

⅛ teaspoon black pepper

Preheat the oven to 350°F.

In a bowl, mix together the flours, butter, egg, and salt. Press the dough evenly into a tart shell, pie dish, or mini tartlet cups. Bake for 10 to 12 minutes if using a tart shell or pie dish, or for 8 to 10 minutes if using a tartlet pan.

Cut the onions in half, and slice very thinly, about ¼ inch thick. In a large pan over low heat, slowly cook the onions for about 40 minutes, until caramelized. Add a small amount of water, as needed, if the onions get too dry.

While the onions are cooking, mix together the DCCC, shredded cheese, egg, salt, and pepper. Refrigerate until ready to use. After the onions have caramelized, spread the cheese filling evenly in the partially baked crust. Spread the onions evenly over the top of the cheese.

Bake for 15 to 20 minutes, or until the center is set. If making tartlets, bake for 8 to 12 minutes. The tart can be wrapped and kept in the refrigerator for up to one week.

Pecan Pie

This pie has a great custard-like texture on the bottom and the crisp crunch of pecans on top. Serve it at Thanksgiving or on a cool winter night with a hot cup of tea.

Makes: 6 to 8 servings

1 Pie Crust (page 110)

2 cups chopped raw pecans

1 tablespoon olive or coconut oil

6 tablespoons (¾ stick) unsalted butter

1 cup Date Paste (page 131)

¾ cup honey

½ teaspoon salt

3 large eggs, room temperature

1 tablespoon pure vanilla extract

¼ cup raw pecan halves, for garnish (optional)

Preheat the oven to 350°F. Prepare the pie crust dough, and roll it out and refrigerate it as described on page 110. Bake the crust for 20 to 25 minutes, until golden brown. Allow to cool.

In a bowl, mix together the chopped pecans and the oil. Spread on a baking sheet, and bake for about 10 minutes, or until lightly browned and fragrant.

While the pecans are toasting, combine the butter, date paste, honey, and salt in a saucepan over medium heat. Bring the mixture to a boil. Remove from the heat, and allow to cool for about 5 minutes.

In a bowl, whisk the eggs. While whisking, pour in a small amount, about ¼ cup, of the butter and date mixture. Combine well, then add an additional ¼ cup, continuing to whisk. Pour in the remaining butter and date mixture, and keep whisking. Stir in the vanilla.

Spread the toasted chopped pecans in the cooled pie crust. Slowly pour the filling over the pecans. Arrange a few pecan halves on top, if desired. Bake for 20 to 25 minutes, or until the center of the pie is set. Allow to cool before serving. The pie can be wrapped and kept in the refrigerator for up to one week.

Almond Pear Tart

Sweet and light, this tart comes together quickly and works with any pear variety. You can even make it with apples if you prefer. Even though the tart is simple, it looks surprisingly sophisticated when finished.

Makes: 6-8 servings

FOR THE PEAR

4 cups water

¼ cup honey

1 tablespoon fresh lemon juice

1 medium pear, peeled, halved, and cored

FOR THE BATTER

¾ cup blanched almond flour

½ cup (1 stick) unsalted butter, room temperature

2 large eggs

1 tablespoon honey

½ teaspoon almond extract

Preheat the oven to 350°F. Prepare a 9-inch tart plate or pie dish by spraying the inside surface with oil or greasing it with butter.

Bring the water, honey, and lemon juice to a simmer in a small pot over medium heat. To the simmering liquid add the pear halves, and cook for 2 to 3 minutes. Remove from the water, and allow to cool. Cut the pear into 10 to 12 slices.

To make the batter, mix together the flour, butter, eggs, honey, and almond extract in a bowl. Pour into the prepared tart shell or pie dish. Arrange the pear slices in the batter. Bake for 20 minutes, or until the edges begin to brown and the center is firm. The tart can be wrapped and kept in the refrigerator for up to one week.

Berry Cobbler

Summer berries and cherries are the best. Why not combine them into one antioxidant-rich dessert? Antioxidants help with cell repair and may help to prevent some cancers. On top of that, berries and cherries are full of vitamins and fiber. Use any combination of summer berries in this recipe.

Makes: 6 to 8 servings

FOR THE FILLING

1 cup dates

4 cups fresh berries and cherries, stems and pits removed

¼ cup (½ stick) unsalted butter, softened

3 tablespoons fresh lemon juice

FOR THE TOPPING

2 cups blanched almond flour

½ teaspoon baking soda

½ teaspoon salt

½ cup SCD Yogurt (page 129)

2 teaspoons lemon zest

Preheat the oven to 375°F. Butter the inside surface of a 9 × 12-inch baking dish.

Soak the dates in hot water until softened, about 15 minutes. Drain the water, and remove the pits. Chop the dates into ¼-inch pieces. In a bowl, mix together the berries and cherries, dates, butter, and lemon juice. Pour the berry mixture into the prepared baking dish.

To make the topping, mix together the flour, baking soda, salt, yogurt, and lemon zest in a separate bowl. Spread the topping evenly over the fruit mixture, covering from edge to edge.

Bake for 20 to 25 minutes, or until the fruit mixture bubbles at the edges and the topping starts to brown. Allow to cool for at least 5 minutes before serving. The cobbler can be covered and kept in the refrigerator for up to one week.

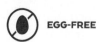 **EGG-FREE**

Blueberry Pie

Blueberries are a powerhouse of vitamins and other nutrients, with one of the highest concentrations of antioxidants of all fruits. You can feel good about eating this pie, even though it is dessert. Nearly all of the sweetness comes from the blueberries, and just a little from honey. This dessert is best enjoyed the same day, as the juicy berries soften the bottom crust after some time.

Makes: 6 to 8 servings

2 Pie Crust (page 110)

6 cups fresh or frozen blueberries

¼ cup honey

1 tablespoon fresh lemon juice

1 teaspoon gelatin powder

1 large egg, beaten

Preheat the oven to 350°F. Prepare the pie crust as described on page 110. Parbake for 10 to 15 minutes.

To make the filling, mix together the blueberries, honey, lemon juice, and gelatin in a pot. Bring to a simmer over low heat, stirring occasionally. Allow to simmer for about 10 minutes. Remove the rolled-out dough, and set aside. Pour the cooked blueberries into the partially baked pie crust. Place the rolled-out dough over the top of the pie, slice off any overhang, and cut three ventilation slits on top. As an alternative, cut the rolled-out dough into strips, and weave a lattice top. Brush the beaten egg on the top crust or lattice topping.

Bake for 15 to 20 minutes, or until the top crust is crisp and golden. Allow to cool for at least 10 minutes before serving. The pie can be wrapped and kept in the refrigerator for two to three days.

Lemon Meringue Pie

With its crisp crust, its creamy and tangy filling, and its pillowy meringue topping, this pie is refreshing and feels a bit decadent to eat. You can adjust the tartness of the filling by increasing or decreasing the amount of lemon zest. Feel free to use other citrus fruits like lime or grapefruit.

Makes: 6 to 8 servings

1 Pie Crust (page 110)

FOR THE FILLING
5 large egg yolks

½ cup fresh lemon juice

¼ cup honey

1 tablespoon lemon zest

¼ cup (½ stick) unsalted butter

FOR THE MERINGUE
¼ cup honey

5 large egg whites, chilled

1 teaspoon fresh lemon juice

Preheat the oven to 350°F. Prepare the pie crust as described on page 110. Bake for 20 to 25 minutes, until golden brown. Allow to cool. Reduce the oven to 325°F.

To make the filling, mix together the egg yolks, lemon juice, honey, lemon zest, and butter in a pot over medium-high heat. Stir until the filling begins to thicken and remove from heat. Pour the filling through a fine-mesh strainer into the cooled pie crust.

To make the meringue, heat the honey in a small pot over medium-low heat. When the mixture begins to simmer, remove it from the heat. In a separate bowl, whip the egg whites until soft peaks form, about 3 to 5 minutes. Slowly add the lemon juice and honey while continuing to whip. Keep whipping until stiff peaks form, another 2 to 3 minutes. Spoon the meringue over the pie filling.

Bake for 12 to 15 minutes, until the meringue is golden brown. Cool to room temperature before serving. The pie can be wrapped and kept in the refrigerator for two to three days.

TIP: To check if your filling is thickening, dip a spoon into the filling and then pull your finger across the spoon, through the filling that has coated it. If it creates a clean line, then your filling is ready.

Coconut Custard Pie

This coconut custard could be a pie filling, but it is so delicious on its own, no crust is needed. Once cooled, this dessert can be sliced and it will hold its shape. The custard is creamy and soft under a crisp coating of coconut.

Makes: 6 to 8 servings

2 cups coconut milk

1 tablespoon coconut flour

½ teaspoon baking soda

¼ teaspoon salt

4 large eggs, room temperature

⅓ cup honey

½ teaspoon pure vanilla extract

½ teaspoon pure coconut extract

1 cup finely grated coconut

Preheat the oven to 350°F. Butter the inside surface of a 9-inch pie dish or cake pan.

Whisk together the milk, flour, baking soda, salt, eggs, honey, and extracts, making sure all ingredients are very well incorporated. Stir in the coconut flakes. Pour the mixture into the prepared dish or pan.

Bake for 25 to 30 minutes, or until the edges have browned and the center is nearly set. Allow to cool slightly before serving. The custard will keep in the refrigerator, covered for up to one week.

Pumpkin Pie

Packed full of vitamins A and E and magnesium as well as other nutrients, pumpkin is a super healthy fruit to include in your diet. This pie filling isn't as custardy as in traditional pumpkin pie, as it doesn't contain sweetened condensed milk. Instead, the filling is smooth and pudding-like.

Makes: 6 to 8 servings

1 Pie Crust (page 110) or Pecan Pie Crust (page 112)

2 cups pure pumpkin puree

2 large eggs

½ cup coconut milk

¼ cup honey

1 teaspoon pure vanilla extract

½ teaspoon ground cinnamon

¼ teaspoon ground ginger

⅛ teaspoon ground cloves

⅛ teaspoon ground nutmeg

Preheat the oven to 350°F. Prepare the pie crust dough according to the instructions on page 110 or page 112. Parbake the crust for 10 to 15 minutes if making the Pie Crust recipe or 5 to 8 minutes if using the Pecan Pie Crust.

In a bowl, mix together the pumpkin, eggs, milk, honey, vanilla, and spices until fully incorporated. Pour into the partially baked pie crust, and cover the edges with foil or a crust protector to prevent burning.

Bake for 40 to 50 minutes, or until the center of the pie has set. Allow to cool slightly before serving. Store covered in the refrigerator for up to one week.

Quiche

No longer for special occasions, quiche is a delectable go-to meal for breakfast, lunch, or dinner. You have a lot of freedom with this recipe, to come up with different fillings. You can make it spicy or mild, and vegetarian or filled with meat. Serve it by itself or with a salad or a cup of soup.

Makes: 6 to 8 servings

1 Savory Pie Crust (page 111)

3 large eggs

1½ cups nut milk or coconut milk

⅛ teaspoon salt

½ teaspoon additional seasonings of choice such as garlic, basil, thyme (optional)

2 cups vegetables, meat, and/or shredded cheese

Preheat the oven to 350°F. Prepare the Savory Pie Crust dough, and roll it out and refrigerate it as described on page 111.

Whisk together the eggs, milk, salt, and seasonings, if using. Sauté the vegetables or cook the meat that will be used. Spread the sautéed vegetables, cooked meat, and cheese evenly in the pie crust. Gently pour the egg mixture on top.

Bake for 25 to 30 minutes, until the center has set. The quiche can be wrapped and kept in the refrigerator for up to one week.

Flavor Suggestions

Spinach, tomato, basil, and Parmesan cheese

Caramelized onions and mushrooms

Broccoli and cheddar cheese

Spinach, bacon, and Swiss cheese

Tomato Pie

This summer favorite features the season's bounty of juicy tomatoes. You can use any tomato variety for this pie. The richness of the mayonnaise and the cheese perfectly balances the acidity of the tomatoes. This pie travels well, so plan on bringing it to a picnic or summer potluck.

Makes: About 6 to 8 servings

1 Savory Pie Crust (page 111)

3 cups sliced tomatoes (3 to 4 large tomatoes)

1½ teaspoons salt

½ cup dry curd cottage cheese (DCCC)

¼ teaspoon black pepper

2 tablespoons fresh basil or 1 teaspoon dried basil

1 small yellow onion, peeled and thinly sliced

½ cup mayonnaise

1½ cups shredded provolone cheese

Preheat the oven to 350°F. Prepare the Savory Pie Crust dough, and roll it out and refrigerate it as described on page 111. Partially bake the pie crust for 10 to 15 minutes.

Slice the tomatoes, lay them on paper towels, and sprinkle with the salt. In a small bowl, mix together the DCCC, pepper, and basil. In a separate bowl, mix together the mayonnaise and the provolone.

Spread the seasoned DCCC over the bottom of the partially baked pie crust. Arrange the onion slices in a single layer on top of the DCCC. Then layer on the tomato slices. Spread the mayonnaise and provolone mixture over the top of the tomatoes. Cover the edges of the crust with foil or a crust protector.

Bake for 30 to 40 minutes, or until the provolone starts to brown Allow to cool slightly before serving. The pie can be wrapped and kept in the refrigerator for up to one week.

Rustic Berry Tart

Sometimes you don't want to bother with a tart shell or pie dish and just want to throw something together, free-form, on a baking sheet. This tart is designed for just such occasion. It is sophisticated without being fussy. The juices may bubble over the sides or through small cracks in the dough. That's part of this tart's charm and rustic appeal.

Makes: About 6 to 8 servings

FOR THE CRUST

½ cup coconut flour

¾ cup blanched almond flour

½ cup (1 stick) unsalted butter, chilled and cut into cubes

1 large egg

2 tablespoons honey

FOR THE FILLING

3 cups fresh berries

¼ cup chopped dates

2 tablespoons butter, chilled and cut into cubes

Preheat the oven to 350°F. Prepare a baking sheet by lining it with parchment paper.

In a food processor, combine all of the ingredients for the crust. Pulse 3 or 4 times, until all of the ingredients have come together. Alternatively, rub together the flours and butter until combined. Stir in the egg and honey. Scrape the dough onto a sheet of plastic wrap. Form the dough into a ball, pat it down a little, then cover it with a second sheet of plastic wrap. Roll the dough into a rough circle, about ¼ inch thick. Slide the plastic-wrap or parchment covered disk onto a large flat surface, such as a cutting board, and place it in the refrigerator for 30 minutes or the freezer for 10 minutes.

In a separate bowl, gently combine the berries, dates, and butter. Remove the rolled-out dough from the refrigerator, take off the top layer of plastic wrap, and transfer the dough to the baking sheet. Allow the dough to warm enough to be pliable, about 2 to 3 minutes. Drain any liquid that may be in with the berries, then pour the berry mixture onto the center of the dough. Carefully fold the edges of the dough over the berries, leaving the center open.

Bake for 15 to 25 minutes, or until golden brown. Allow to cool slightly before serving. This tart is best enjoyed the same day it is made.

Cranberry Apple Crisp

For the best texture and flavor, use a variety of apples, such as Honeycrisp, Golden Delicious, and Rome. As this crisp bakes, it fills your home with the sweet smell of cinnamon and makes you think of autumn.

Makes: 4 to 6 servings

FOR THE FILLING

¼ cup dried, unsweetened cranberries

4 medium apples

1 teaspoon ground cinnamon

2 tablespoons honey

FOR THE TOPPING

¼ cup blanched almond flour

¼ cup coconut flour

1 tablespoon unsalted butter

¼ cup chopped almonds

¼ teaspoon ground cinnamon

⅛ teaspoon salt

Preheat the oven to 350 °F. Butter the inside of a 7-inch by 11-inch baking dish.

Soak the cranberries in hot water for 5 minutes. While the cranberries are soaking, peel and core the apples, then cut into ½-inch slices. In a bowl, combine the drained cranberries, apple slices, cinnamon, and honey. Place the apple filling into the prepared baking dish.

In a separate bowl, combine the flours with the butter, using your fingers until the mixture is combined and has the consistency of sand. Add the almonds, cinnamon, and salt, mixing until well combined. Spread the topping evenly over the filling.

Bake for 30 to 40 minutes, or until the topping is browned. Allow to cool for about 10 minutes before serving. The crisp can be wrapped and kept in the refrigerator for up to one week.

 EGG-FREE

Pastry-Covered Baked Apples

Warm and comforting, one of these baked apples is like a single-serving apple pie. Use Gala, Honeycrisp, Cortland, Pink Lady, or other firm apple variety that will hold its shape during baking. A fun variation of this recipe is to fill the cored center of the apple with dried fruit and nuts before baking.

Makes: 3 servings

FOR THE PASTRY

1 cup blanched almond flour

¼ cup coconut flour

¼ teaspoon baking soda

⅓ cup (⅔ stick) unsalted butter, room temperature

1 large egg, room temperature

3 tablespoons honey

½ teaspoon ground cinnamon

FOR THE APPLES

3 medium apples, peeled and cored

1 tablespoon unsalted butter

1 teaspoon ground cinnamon

Preheat the oven to 350ºF. Line a baking sheet with parchment paper.

To make the pastry, thoroughly combine the flours, baking soda, butter, egg, honey, and cinnamon in a large bowl.

To prepare the apples, divide the butter and cinnamon into thirds, and place them in the cored centers of the apples.

Lay down a piece of plastic wrap, put a third of the pastry dough in the center, and place a second piece of plastic wrap on top. Using a rolling pin, roll the dough until ¼ inch thick. Remove the top layer of plastic wrap, and place an apple in the center of the dough. Fold the dough up over the apple, covering all sides. Pinch or press the dough together if small tears appear. Repeat with the remaining apples.

Bake for 25 to 30 minutes, or until the crust is browned.

Pie Crust

This is the recipe that I used to make all of the dessert pies in this book. It holds its shape when a slice is lifted out of a pie plate and is a good base for the various fillings.

Makes: One 9-inch pie crust

½ cup coconut flour

½ cup blanched almond flour

½ cup (1 stick) unsalted butter, chilled and cut into cubes

1 large egg, room temperature

In a food processor, combine all of the ingredients. Pulse three or four times, until they all come together. Alternatively, you can use your fingers to rub the flours, salt, and butter together until combined, then stir in the egg. For a very smooth and even crust, scrape the dough onto a large piece of plastic wrap or parchment paper. Place another piece of plastic wrap or parchment paper on top of the dough, and roll it into a disk shape ¼ inch thick and about 11 to 12 inches in diameter. Slide the plastic-wrap or parchment covered disk onto a large flat surface, such as a cutting board, and place it in the refrigerator for 30 minutes or the freezer for 10 minutes.

If the dough becomes too cold, allow it to warm slightly so that it is pliable enough to form to the pie dish. Flip the dough over onto the pie dish, and gently press down. Trim any overhanging dough and use it to fill any cracks. For a more rustic crust, you may use your fingers to press the dough into the pie dish until it is evenly distributed and covers the bottom and sides.

To partially bake the crust, place it in a 350°F oven for 10 to 15 minutes, until the crust begins to firm up. Bake for 20 to 25 minutes if using a filling that does not require further baking, such as custard.

TIP: If you want a dryer, less buttery crust, reduce the amount of butter by as much as ¼ cup.

Savory Pie Crust

This pie crust is the same as the pie crust used for the dessert pies, but has the addition of salt. Use this recipe for quiches and other types of pies containing savory fillings.

Makes: One 9-inch pie crust

½ cup blanched almond flour

½ cup coconut flour

½ cup (1 stick) unsalted butter, chilled and cut into cubes

1 large egg, room temperature

½ teaspoon salt

In a food processor, combine all of the ingredients. Pulse three or four times, until they come together. Alternatively, you can use your fingers to rub the flours, salt, and butter together until combined, then stir in the egg. For a very smooth and even crust, scrape the dough onto a large piece of plastic wrap or parchment paper. Place another piece of plastic wrap or parchment paper on top of the dough, and roll it into a disk shape ¼ inch thick and about 11 to 12 inches in diameter. Slide the plastic-wrapped disk onto a large flat surface, such as a cutting board, and place it in the refrigerator for 30 minutes or the freezer for 10 minutes.

If the dough becomes too cold, allow it to warm slightly so that it is pliable enough to form to the pie dish. Flip the dough over onto the pie dish, and gently press the dough down. Trim any overhanging dough and use it to fill in any cracks. For a more rustic crust, you may use your fingers to press the dough into the pie dish until it is evenly distributed and covers the bottom and sides.

To partially bake the crust, place it in a 350°F oven for 10 to 15 minutes, until the crust begins to firm up.

TIP: If you want a dryer, less buttery crust, reduce the amount of butter by as much as ¼ cup.

Pecan Pie Crust

This is the perfect crust for custard-based pies. The nutty crunch contrasts nicely with the smooth custard filling. The crust is especially delicious in pumpkin pie, but feel free to experiment with other pie fillings. This recipe works just as well with other whole nuts, such as cashews and almonds.

Makes: One 9-inch pie crust

2 cups raw pecans

¼ cup (½ stick) unsalted butter, softened

¼ cup Date Paste (page 131)

Preheat the oven to 350°F.

In a food processor, pulse the pecans until they become coarse meal. Add the butter and date paste to the pecans, and pulse until well combined. Alternately, if you don't have a food processor, chop the pecans until they form very coarse meal. Thoroughly mix in the butter and date paste. Press the pecan mixture into a pie plate.

Bake in the oven for 5 to 8 minutes, or until the pecans are fragrant.

Chapter 5
Custards and Soufflés

Baked Caramel Custard

This dessert is similar to Spanish flan, which is usually made with evaporated milk and caramelized sugar. Instead, it uses coconut or nut milk and caramelized honey.

Makes: Four 6-ounce ramekins

¾ cup honey, divided

2 cups Coconut Milk (page 130) or Nut Milk (page 128)

3 large eggs

1 teaspoon pure vanilla extract

⅛ teaspoon salt

Preheat the oven to 350°F.

In a small pot or pan over medium-high heat, heat ½ cup of the honey until it boils. Let it boil for about 3 to 5 minutes, then pour it into four 6-ounce ramekins. In a bowl, whisk together the remaining honey, milk, eggs, vanilla, and salt. Divide the milk mixture evenly among the ramekins.

Place the ramekins in a baking dish, and add about an inch of hot water to the dish. Carefully place the baking dish in the oven. Bake for 40 to 45 minutes, or until only the center of the custard wobbles when shaken. Allow to cool in the refrigerator before serving.

Chai Custard

This baked custard tastes like chai tea, even though there isn't any tea in the recipe. All of the flavor comes from the same spices used in making chai tea.

Makes: Six 4-ounce ramekins

1½ cups Coconut Milk (page 130) or Nut Milk (page 128)

¼ cup honey

3 cardamom pods, crushed

1 stick cinnamon or ⅛ teaspoon ground cinnamon

4 cloves or ⅛ teaspoon ground cloves

⅛ teaspoon ground ginger

3 large eggs

Preheat the oven to 350°F.

In a pot over medium heat, heat the milk with the honey, cardamom, cinnamon, cloves, and ginger. Bring to a simmer, turn off the heat, and allow the spices to steep for 5 to 10 minutes. After steeping, pour through a fine-mesh strainer into a bowl. In a separate bowl, whisk the eggs while slowly pouring in the warm spiced milk. Divide the mixture among the ramekins.

Place the ramekins in a baking dish, and add about an inch of hot water to the dish. Gently place the baking dish in the oven. Bake for 20 to 25 minutes, or until the center of the custard has set. Allow to cool in the water bath for 15 to 20 minutes before serving.

Honey Crème Brûlée

Sweet and creamy with a crisp crust to crack through, crème brûlée is a fancy dessert that you can play with. There is something so devilish about breaking through that crisp caramelized crust! This dessert does take some time, since the custard needs to cool completely before the top can be brûléed, so plan ahead. The recipe calls for coconut cream for its flavor and fat content, but coconut milk can be used if coconut cream isn't available. Make sure to have a kitchen torch on hand or a broiler to brûlée, or caramelize, the honey.

Makes: Eight 6-ounce ramekins

4 cups Coconut Cream (page 130)

⅓ cup honey, plus more for brûlée

6 large egg yolks

1 tablespoon pure vanilla extract

Preheat the oven to 325°F.

Whisk together the coconut cream, honey, egg yolks, and vanilla. Divide the mixture among eight 6-ounce ramekins.

Place the ramekins in a baking dish, and add about an inch of hot water to the dish. Gently place the baking dish in the oven. Bake for 30 to 40 minutes, or until the center of the custard is just set. Remove the custards, and cool in the refrigerator for a minimum of 45 minutes.

Once the custards have cooled, remove them from the refrigerator. Add a thin layer of honey to the top of each custard. Using a kitchen torch, brûlée the honey until it bubbles and turns golden brown. Place the custards back in the refrigerator for an additional 30 minutes before serving.

Cherry Clafouti

Clafouti is a light fruit custard that forms a crust as it bakes. It is one of those desserts that is both rustic and elegant. This version has a delicate sweetness, with cherries hidden in every bite. Everyone will be amazed by your baking prowess when you place this dessert on the table.

Makes: 6 to 8 servings

1 tablespoon unsalted butter or coconut oil, room temperature

3 large eggs

4 tablespoons honey, divided

1 ¼ cup Nut Milk (page 128) or Coconut Milk (page 130)

¼ cup plus 2 tablespoons blanched almond flour

2 teaspoons pure vanilla extract

¼ teaspoon salt

1 cup pitted cherries

SCD Yogurt (page 129) (optional)

mint sprig, for garnish (optional)

Preheat the oven to 350°F. Butter or oil the bottom of a 9 × 13-inch baking dish.

Whisk together the eggs and 2 tablespoons of the honey until light in color. Add the milk, flour, vanilla, and salt, mixing until fully integrated. Drizzle the remaining 2 tablespoons of honey into the baking dish. Spread the cherries evenly in the dish, and very slowly pour in the batter, careful not to disturb the cherries.

Bake for 35 to 45 minutes, or until the custard is firm and golden. Serve warm, adding a dollop of SCD Yogurt and a sprig of mint if desired.

Meringue-Covered Peaches

These peaches are clothed in a billowy cloud of meringue. They are extra delicious served with Fruit Sauce, page 127.

Makes: 4 servings

4 large egg whites, chilled

1 teaspoon fresh lemon juice or white vinegar

2 tablespoons honey

4 medium peaches, cut in half, pits removed

Heat the oven to 350°F. Line a baking sheet with parchment paper.

In a bowl, whip the egg whites and lemon juice or vinegar until stiff peaks form. In a small saucepan over medium heat, heat the honey to a boil. Allow the honey to boil for about 1 minute. With the mixer on, slowly drizzle the hot honey into the egg whites and mix until the honey is just incorporated. Put the two halves of each peach back together. Spoon a small amount of the meringue onto the baking sheet, then place the peaches on top. Spoon the remaining meringue over the peaches, covering all surfaces of the fruit.

Bake for 15 to 20 minutes, until the meringue is golden.

Bread Pudding

Comfort food at its best, bread pudding is a satisfying way to use up leftover bread and bread heels. It is okay to mix different breads—for example, the Sandwich Bread (page 14), Banana Bread (page 21), and Peach Bread (page 28) go really well together. The pudding is yummy with the warm Date Sauce on page 120 or Fruit Sauce, page 127, served on top.

Makes: 6 to 8 servings

4 large eggs

2 cups Nut Milk (page 128) or Coconut Milk (page 130)

¼ cup honey

1 teaspoon pure vanilla extract

1 teaspoon ground cinnamon

6 cups bread, cut into 1-inch cubes

½ cup raisins or other dried fruit (optional)

Preheat the oven to 350°F. Prepare a 9 by 13-inch baking dish by greasing it with butter or lining it with parchment paper.

In a bowl, mix together the eggs, milk, honey, vanilla, and cinnamon. Soak the bread cubes in the egg mixture. Place half of the bread cubes in the baking dish, sprinkle on half of the raisins or other dried fruit, if using, and add the remaining bread cubes and top with raisins or dried fruit. Bake for 40 to 45 minutes, until the eggs are set and the bread is golden. Serve warm or at room temperature. Store covered in the refrigerator for up to one week.

Sticky Toffee Pudding

Warm, sweet, and comforting, sticky toffee pudding is a traditional British dessert made with dates. It is usually served with toffee sauce, ordinarily made with sugar and heavy cream, but this version uses date syrup and SCD Yogurt. If you have never tried sticky toffee pudding, I highly recommend whipping up this recipe.

Makes: 6 to 8 servings

FOR THE PUDDING

1¼ cups pitted dates, chopped, divided

¾ cup hot water

¾ cup blanched almond flour

1½ teaspoons baking soda

½ teaspoon salt

½ cup honey

2 large eggs

1 teaspoon pure vanilla extract

¼ cup (½ stick) unsalted butter, melted

FOR THE DATE SAUCE

½ cup (1 stick) unsalted butter

½ cup date syrup

½ cup SCD Yogurt (page 129)

Preheat the oven to 350°F. Prepare a 9-inch round or square baking dish by buttering or oiling the bottom and sides of the dish.

Pour the hot water over half of the dates. Allow them to soak for 10 to 15 minutes to soften. Meanwhile, whisk together the flour, baking soda, and salt in a bowl. In a food processor, combine the other half of the dates and the honey, processing until smooth. Drain the soaked dates, saving the liquid, and set aside the dates. Add the soaking liquid, eggs, and vanilla to the honey mixture. Process until smooth. Pour the wet mixture, the soaked dates, and melted butter into the flour mixture, and stir to combine.

Pour the batter into the prepared baking dish, and cover with foil. Bake for 30 to 40 minutes, or until slightly puffed and firm to the touch. Allow to cool for about 10 minutes before serving warm with sauce.

For the sauce, melt the butter with the date syrup in a saucepan over medium heat until the edges begin to bubble. Allow to cook for 1 minute longer, then remove from the heat. Whisk in the yogurt, and serve with the warm cake.

Fruit Soufflé

A soufflé can seem intimidating at first, but give this recipe a try and you will find out how simple it is. Light and airy, a soufflé makes a delicious finish to any meal. Serve it with a little Fruit Sauce (page 127) on the side.

Makes: Six 6-ounce ramekins

4 large egg whites

1 teaspoon fresh lemon juice or white vinegar

¼ cup honey

¾ cup fruit, pureed

¼ cup blanched almond flour

Preheat the oven to 350ºF. Place a 9 × 13-inch baking dish filled with 2 cups of hot water on the lower shelf of the oven. Prepare the ramekins by spraying them with vegetable oil.

Whip the egg whites and lemon juice or vinegar until stiff peaks form. In a small saucepan or pot over medium-high heat, bring the honey to a boil. Allow it to boil for 1 minute. With the mixer on, slowly drizzle the hot honey into the egg whites. Whip only until the honey is incorporated. The egg whites will become smoother and glisten slightly.

In a separate bowl, add the pureed fruit. Add 2 heaping spoonfuls of the whipped egg whites into the fruit puree, and stir it in. Add the remaining egg whites, and sift the almond flour on top. Gently fold the egg whites and the almond flour into the fruit puree mixture.

Spoon the batter into the ramekins until three-quarters full. Run your finger or a clean dish towel around the edge of the ramekin, cleaning the rim. Place the ramekins in the baking dish of water. Bake for about 20 minutes, until the soufflés have risen and are slightly browned. Carefully remove from the oven, and serve immediately.

Chapter 6
Frostings and Sauces

Basic Buttercream Frosting

This frosting is smooth, creamy, and a bit reminiscent of cream cheese frosting. It is thick enough to use with a piping bag and as decorative writing on a cake.

Makes: About 3 cups*

1 cup (2 sticks) unsalted butter, room temperature

¾ cup SCD Yogurt (page 129)

¼ cup honey

1 tablespoon pure vanilla extract

In a bowl, whip the butter on medium speed for about 2 to 3 minutes until it becomes very light in color. Add the yogurt, honey, and vanilla, continuing to mix.

Use the frosting right away or refrigerate it for up to a week. If refrigerating, allow the frosting to come to room temperature and then rewhip it to the right consistency. After decorating the cake or cupcakes, refrigerate them until ready to serve.

*2 cups of frosting is enough for one dozen cupcakes or a single-layer 9-inch cake. 3 cups of frosting is enough to cover a double-layer 9-inch cake. The frosting recipes are easily doubled or divided to meet your needs.

Variation

Use almond, lemon, or coconut extract in place of the vanilla extract.

 EGG-FREE

Cocoa Butter Frosting

Who doesn't love chocolate? While this isn't exactly chocolate, it does give baked goods a hint of chocolaty-ness. It complements Peanut Butter Cake (page 55) and Banana Bread (page 21) amazingly well.

Makes: About 2 cups*

½ cup cocoa butter, melted

½ cup (1 stick) unsalted butter, softened

¼ cup honey

1 teaspoon pure vanilla extract

Place the melted cocoa butter in the refrigerator, allowing it to set a little. It should be the same consistency as the softened butter. Once the cocoa butter has reached the right consistency, combine it with the butter in a bowl. Whip until light and fluffy, about 3 to 5 minutes. Drizzle in the honey and vanilla, continuing to whip. Use the frosting right away or refrigerate it for up to a week. If refrigerating, allow the frosting to come to room temperature and then rewhip it to the right consistency. After decorating the cake or cupcakes, refrigerate them until ready to serve.

*2 cups of frosting is enough for one dozen cupcakes or a single-layer 9-inch cake. 3 cups of frosting is enough to cover a double-layer 9-inch cake. The frosting recipes are easily doubled or divided to meet your needs.

TIP: The cocoa butter may harden if the butter is too cold, and this will result in small cocoa butter chips in your frosting. It is still delicious to use this way.

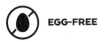 EGG-FREE

Banana Frosting

Have too many overripe bananas? Use a couple in this frosting for spreading on cookies, cakes, and even some breads. It is excellent on Peanut Butter Cake (page 55), Peanut Butter Banana Muffins (page 54), Banana Bread (page 21), and on the Vanilla Shortbread Cookies (page 82).

Makes: About 2 cups*

½ cup (1 stick) unsalted butter, softened

2 large very ripe bananas

1 tablespoon honey

½ teaspoon pure vanilla extract

Whip the butter until light and fluffy, about 2 to 3 minutes. Add the bananas, honey, and vanilla, and continue to whip until well combined Use the frosting right away or refrigerate it for up to a week. If refrigerating, allow the frosting to come to room temperature and then rewhip it to the right consistency. After decorating the cake or cupcakes, refrigerate them until ready to serve.

*2 cups of frosting is enough for one dozen cupcakes or a single-layer 9-inch cake. 3 cups of frosting is enough to cover a double-layer 9-inch cake. The frosting recipes are easily doubled or divided to meet your needs.

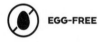 **EGG-FREE**

Fruit Sauce

Pour this sauce over nearly any dessert to add sweetness and color. For the best flavor, take advantage of fruit that is in season. Ripe fruit that is in season will be sweeter and will need less honey than out of season fruit.

Makes: About 1½ cups

2 cups fresh or thawed frozen fruit   2 tablespoons to ¼ cup honey

Cut up the fruit, and place in a blender. Blend until pureed, about 1 to 2 minutes. Transfer the pureed fruit to a saucepan over medium-low heat. Add honey until the desired sweetness is reached. Bring the fruit sauce to a simmer, stirring to prevent burning. Serve hot or chilled.

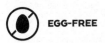 EGG-FREE

TIP: For a smoother sauce, strain the fruit after pureeing it.

Appendix: Essential SCD Recipes

Nut Milk

The uses for nut milk are endless—I use it in cakes, cookies, custards, yogurt, and sauces. If you prefer a creamier milk, add more nuts. This recipe can be made with almost any variety of nut, such as almonds, cashews, or pecans.

Makes: 4 cups

1½ to 3 cups nuts

6½ cups filtered water, divided

1 teaspoon pure vanilla extract (optional)

3 dates, pitted (optional)

In a medium bowl, cover the nuts with 2 cups of the filtered water. Allow the nuts to soak for 10 to 12 hours, or overnight. Drain the soaking water, and rinse the nuts.

Place the soaked nuts in a blender, and add the remaining 4½ cups of filtered water along with the vanilla and dates, if using. Blend for 2 to 4 minutes, or until completely blended. Through several layers of cheesecloth or a nut milk bag, drain the nut mixture into a bowl. Gently squeeze the mixture to release all of the remaining moisture. Pour the nut milk from the bowl into an airtight a container.

The nut milk will keep for one week in the refrigerator. Shake before serving.

TIP: The nut meal that remains in the cheesecloth or nut milk bag can be used in baking. Spread the nut meal out evenly onto a baking sheet lined with parchment paper and dry it in the oven on low heat, around 200°F, for 2 to 3 hours. Freeze it until you are ready to dry it in the oven. Once dried, store it in an airtight container in the refrigerator or freezer.

SCD Yogurt

Yogurt is a very important part of the recovery process on SCD. Many baking recipes call for yogurt as an ingredient, as it gives baked goods a lighter texture and helps activate the baking soda. You can use dairy products (cow's or goat's) or non-dairy nut milk or coconut milk. This recipe uses a yogurt maker, which is just one of the many methods available for making yogurt. Other methods include using a heating pad, or using a slow cooker, or the heat from your oven light. You can purchase a yogurt maker online or at a superstore, such as Target or Kohl's.

Makes: 4 cups

4 cups milk, half and half, or heavy cream, or nut milk or coconut milk

1 teaspoon gelatin (optional, for thicker yogurt)

⅛ teaspoon yogurt starter, such as Yogourmet, or 1½ tablespoons plain, bifidus-free yogurt

In a saucepan over medium-low heat, heat the milk, half and half, or heavy cream to 180°F, stirring to avoid curdling or burning. Remove from the heat, and let cool to 100 to 110°F. Stir in the yogurt starter or yogurt and the gelatin, if using, and transfer to a yogurt maker. Allow yogurt made from dairy products to culture for 24 hours at 110°F. Yogurt made from nut milk or coconut milk needs less time, as little as 12 hours, but up to 24 hours at 110°F. Check the temperature with a thermometer every few hours. Remove the lid of the yogurt maker if the yogurt's temperature climbs above 115°F.

The yogurt can be stored in an airtight container in the refrigerator for up to one week.

Coconut Milk

Many of the recipes in this book call for coconut milk, which gives baked goods a richer flavor and a good texture. It can be difficult to find pure coconut milk in stores; good thing it is so easy to make at home.

Makes: 5 to 6 cups

6 cups unsweetened coconut flakes or 2 whole coconuts   6 cups filtered hot water

If using coconut flakes: Soak the coconut flakes in the hot water for 10 to 15 minutes, then place in a blender and blend on high for 3 to 5 minutes. Drain the milk through cheesecloth or a nut bag set in a strainer. Gently squeeze the mixture to release all of the remaining moisture.

If using whole coconuts: Drill holes into the three circles, or eyes, on the coconut, and drain the liquid. Place the coconuts in a 350°F oven for 5 minutes. With a hammer, tap around the coconut until it splits open. Using a spoon or a butter knife, remove the white coconut meat. Use a vegetable peeler or paring knife to remove any brown husk that remains on the meat. Soak the cleaned coconut meat in the hot water for 10 to 15 minutes, then blend for 3 to 5 minutes. Drain the milk through cheesecloth or a nut bag set in a strainer. Gently squeeze the mixture to release all of the remaining moisture.

Pour the coconut milk from the bowl into an airtight a container.

The coconut milk will keep for one week in the refrigerator. Shake before serving.

Coconut Cream

To make coconut cream, just refrigerate coconut milk for 12 to 24 hours. The cream will rise to the top. Scoop it out to separate it from the milk. The coconut milk recipe above will give you ¼ to ½ cup of cream.

Date Paste

Dates have been used as a sweetener for thousands of years. In addition to being a good source of potassium, they are rich in fiber. This date paste is very versatile in that it can be eaten as a spread, mixed in dips, or used to sweeten baked goods. It's so yummy, with a slightly fruity brown sugar flavor.

Makes: About 1½ cups

2 cups pitted whole dates   3 cups water

In a pot over medium heat, bring the dates and the water to a simmer. Allow to simmer for a couple of minutes, and then turn off the heat. Let the dates soak for 10 to 15 minutes. Drain the water, saving it in a separate bowl. Place the dates in a blender, and blend until smooth. Add a little of the soaking water if needed for a very smooth paste. Refrigerate for up to one week in an airtight container.

TIP: Save the leftover soaking water, which contains some nutrients and sweetness, to use in smoothies or to stir into yogurt.

Extracts

A great way to add flavor without adding a lot of liquid, extracts are incredibly easy to make. They require very few ingredients and very little work. As an added bonus, they can be stored at room temperature indefinitely, as the alcohol is a preservative. Make sure to use sterile jars to steep and store the extracts. Any of these flavors would be yummy additions to frostings or nut milk.

Vanilla Extract

6 to 8 vanilla beans
1 cup vodka

Slice the vanilla beans in half lengthwise, and place in a glass jar with a lid. Pour the vodka over the vanilla beans, and close the lid. Allow to steep for a minimum of three months in a cool, dark place, shaking every week or so. The beans may remain in the extract or may be removed after the three months. Store in a cool, dark place.

Coffee Extract

¼ cup coffee beans
1 cup vodka

Place the coffee beans and vodka in a blender. Pulse several times, until the beans are ground and the mixture is very dark. Strain out the ground coffee beans using cheesecloth, a coffee filter, or a nut bag, and pour the extract into a glass container with a lid. For an even stronger extract, leave the ground beans in the vodka for several days before straining. Store in a cool, dark place.

Orange or Lemon Extract

Peel from 1 large orange or 2 medium lemons
1 cup vodka

With a paring knife, carefully remove the white pith on the orange peel, as it will make the extract bitter. Place the cleaned peel in a glass jar with a lid, and cover with the vodka. Close the lid, and let steep for about 1 month in a cool, dark place, shaking every couple of days. Remove the peels and store in a cool, dark place.

Almond Extract

¼ cup chopped blanched almonds
1 cup vodka

Place the almonds in a glass jar with a lid. Pour the vodka over the almonds, and close the lid. Allow to steep for a minimum of three months in a cool, dark place, shaking every week or so. After three months, strain out the almonds, and store in a cool, dark place.

Coconut Extract

¼ cup shredded fresh or dried coconut
¼ to ⅓ cup vodka

Combine the coconut and the vodka in a glass jar with a lid. Add just enough vodka to completely cover the coconut. Allow to steep for three months in a cool dark place, shaking a couple of times per week. After three months, strain the mixture, and store the extract in a cool, dark place.

Conversions

Temperature Conversions

Fahrenheit (°F)	Celsius (°C)
325°F	165°C
350°F	175°C
375°F	190°C
400°F	200°C
425°F	220°C
450°F	230°C

Volume Conversions

U.S.	U.S. equivalent	Metric
1 tablespoon (3 teaspoons)	½ fluid ounce	15 milliliters
¼ cup	2 fluid ounces	60 milliliters
⅓ cup	3 fluid ounces	90 milliliters
½ cup	4 fluid ounces	120 milliliters
⅔ cup	5 fluid ounces	150 milliliters
¾ cup	6 fluid ounces	180 milliliters
1 cup	8 fluid ounces	240 milliliters
2 cups	16 fluid ounces	480 milliliters

Weight Conversions

U.S.	Metric
½ ounce	15 grams
1 ounce	30 grams
2 ounces	60 grams
¼ pound	115 grams
⅓ pound	150 grams
½ pound	225 grams
¾ pound	350 grams
1 pound	450 grams

Recipe Index

About the Author

Kathryn Anible lives an exciting life as a personal chef cooking for people in their homes and by creating beautiful food for catered events. She loves to nourish people, and her favorite pastime is throwing dinner parties for friends. Kathryn studied culinary arts and nutrition at Johnson and Wales University and has always found the science of food and cooking fascinating. She focuses on cooking for specialty diets and finds great pleasure in making her clients, as well as her friends, happy through their bellies.

She also wrote *The Leafy Greens Cookbook* (Ulysses Press, 2013).